UNDERSTANDING MENTAL DISTRESS

Knowledge, Practice and Neoliberal Reform in Community Mental Health Services

Rich Moth

First published in Great Britain in 2022 by

Policy Press, an imprint of
Bristol University Press
University of Bristol
1-9 Old Park Hill
Bristol
BS2 8BB
UK
t: +44 (0)117 954 5940
e: bup-info@bristol.ac.uk

Details of international sales and distribution partners are available at
policy.bristoluniversitypress.co.uk

British Library Cataloguing in Publication Data
A catalogue record for this book is available from the British Library

ISBN 978-1-4473-4987-7 hardcover
ISBN 978-1-4473-4990-7 ePub
ISBN 978-1-4473-4988-4 ePdf

Cover design: Qube Design
Front cover image: GettyImages-698892680 (1)
Bristol University Press and Policy Press use environmentally responsible
print partners.
Printed in Great Britain by CPI Group (UK) Ltd, Croydon, CR0 4YY

Dedicated to the memory of my grandparents, Patricia and
George Williams

Contents

List of tables

List of abbreviations

A&E	Accident & Emergency
AMHP	Approved mental health professional
CBT	Cognitive behavioural therapy
CMHN	Community mental health nurse
CMHT	Community Mental Health Team
COHSE	Confederation of Health Service Employees
CPA	Care Programme Approach
CQUIN	Commissioning for Quality and Innovation
CTO	Community treatment order
DSM	*Diagnostic and Statistical Manual of Mental Disorders*
EIS	Early Intervention Service
EM	Emergentist Marxism
FTE	Full-time equivalent
GP	General practitioner
HoNOS	Health of the Nation Outcome Scales
ICT	Information and communication technology
KPI	Key performance indicator
LGBTQ	Lesbian, gay, bisexual, transgender and queer
M/M	Morphogenetic/morphostatic model
MHA	Mental Health Act
MHPS	Mental Health Payments System
MP	Member of Parliament
NHS	National Health Service
NPM	New Public Management
OAP	Out-of-area placement
PbR	Payment by Results
PICU	Psychiatric intensive care unit
RCN	Royal College of Nursing
RD	Revolving door
RRT	Rehabilitation and Recovery Team
SLM	Service-line management
ST5/SpR	Specialty registrar (psychiatrist)
UK	United Kingdom

Notes on the author

Rich Moth is Senior Lecturer in Social Work at the School of Social Sciences, Liverpool Hope University, UK. Before moving into social work education, he worked for 15 years in various roles in the social care sector, including as a mental health social worker. Rich has worked alongside activists from the survivor and disabled people's movements as an ally in a number of mental health, welfare and anti-austerity campaigns. He is a longstanding member of the national steering committee of the Social Work Action Network (SWAN) and an active trade unionist.

Acknowledgements

I would like to begin by acknowledging an enormous debt of gratitude to the practitioners, service users and carers linked to the 'Southville' Community Mental Health Team (CMHT) and Rehabilitation and Recovery Team (RRT) for their support for and engagement with this study, despite the significant pressures faced by all, and for making me feel welcome during the fieldwork.

This book emerged out of and built on my PhD thesis completed at the University of Birmingham. I am particularly grateful to my initial lead supervisor, Ann Davis, for seeing the potential in the study, and for her crucial role in helping me to access PhD studentship funding. This was initially through the Centre of Excellence in Interdisciplinary Mental Health (CEIMH) at the University of Birmingham, and then through a studentship from the Economic and Social Research Council (ESRC) (grant number ES/ I901817/1). Ann has more recently offered me encouragement and support to write up this monograph, for which I am extremely grateful. I would also like to thank my other PhD supervisors: Jerry Tew, who offered expertise, insight and continuity over the five years (and was extremely helpful with the ESRC application); and Sue White for her great theoretical clarity and ethnographer's insight. Thanks also to CEIMH and the ESRC for their invaluable financial support. In addition, I would like to thank my PhD examiners David Pilgrim and Denise Tanner, for very useful discussion during the Viva and for encouraging advice and feedback.

Expressions of gratitude to two scholars who are, sadly, no longer with us are also important and necessary. Roy Bhaskar generously offered feedback on some draft sections of my PhD thesis and some very helpful comments after its completion. Also, Geoff Pearson offered supervisory input, and extremely beneficial advice as my MA dissertation supervisor at Goldsmiths College, University of London (my MA dissertation was an early iteration of this project).

Activists in social movements have been a source of great inspiration both for the book and in a wider political sense. Particular thanks go to colleagues past and present from campaigning network the Social Work Action Network (SWAN), including Michael Lavalette, Iain Ferguson, Laura Penketh, Vasilios Ioakimidis, Alissa Ruane, Dan Morton, Barrie Levine, Linda Harms-Smith, Jeremy Weinstein, Malcolm Jones, Mark Baldwin, Rea Maglajlic, Terry Murphy, Simon Cardy, Nick Burke, Andy Brammer, Des McDermott and Jo McLaughlin. I would also like to give a particular mention to friends and colleagues from the service user/survivor and disabled people's movements for the inspiration they have provided, including Guy Jamieson, Trish Stoll, Carys McKenna, Peter Beresford, Denise McKenna, Paula Peters, Liz Epps,

Bob Williams-Findlay, Ellen Clifford, Anne O'Donnell and Rick Burgess as well as wider allies in radical mental health activism – Helen Spandler, Mick McKeown, Phil Thomas, Mal Kinney, Paul Atkinson and Beth Greenhill.

I would like to extend thanks for friendship and support to my colleagues at Liverpool Hope University – Scott Massie, Kellie Thompson, Rose Devereux, Nicki Blundell, Philomena Harrison, Amina Saeed, Steven Lucas, Hakan Acar and Wendy Coxshall – and to members of the SUGaH (the Service User and carer Group at Hope). Thanks also to fellow University and College Union activists – Noreen O'Sullivan, Rhona O'Brien, Dave Neary and Lucy Hanson – for friendship and comradeship in the struggle!

I am extremely grateful to many dear friends who have influenced my thinking over the years through our chats about work (and sometimes activism) in mental health and wider welfare services: Stefan Wiese, Steve Sincock, Dave Wileman, Jo Quinlan, Jonny Voss, Caoimhe O'Sullivan, Alan McCormick, Kerry Gallagher, Naz Bharwani, Daphna Rosanis, Lee Murphy, Mark McEvoy, Jon Woods, Jenny Woods, Laura Meehan and Tarin Unwin. A particular shout out and thanks also to Emily Hart and Joe Greener, close friends, fellow activists and co-authors with whom I've explored and developed my analysis of the (punitive) politics of the welfare state in recent years!

My sincere thanks go to the team at Policy Press, Isobel Bainton and Emma Cook, and at various points Helen Davis and Sarah Bird, for their understanding of the many challenges and delays in completing this monograph, and for their help and support along the way.

Before completing this list, some special mentions are needed.

I would like to express enormous thanks to Jonathan Neale and Nancy Lindisfarne, deeply valued friends and comrades, whose confidence in me gave me the impetus I needed to first apply to do an undergraduate degree when in my late 20s, and who have long been an incredible source of support and wisdom in academic as in many other matters. I would like to acknowledge a particular debt of gratitude to Jonathan, both for encouraging me to write and publish this book, and for giving me a great deal of assistance with editing and proofreading. His advice and encouragement have been invaluable and significantly improved the book.

Finally, love and thanks to my family, including mum and Kirstin. But, in particular, to Patricia and George Williams, my much missed grandparents, who were there when it mattered. Their memory still burns brightly.

And last but not least, to my son Lucas and my partner Nicola. To Lucas, with all my love, and apologies for any distractions from play caused by this book! And to Nicola – for love, care, forbearance, always being there, tolerating the pressures, and supporting me through all the ups and downs over the long years of conducting the study and writing this book. Thank you both with all my heart.

Acknowledgement of previously published sections

This monograph is, in part, based on my unpublished PhD thesis (Moth, 2014). Sections of Chapter 2 are based on material already published as Moth, R. (2020) 'The business end': neoliberal policy reforms and biomedical residualism in frontline community mental health practice in England. Competition and Change, 24(2): 133–153. Sections of Chapters 1 and 8 are based on a forthcoming paper: Moth, R. (forthcoming a) Sedimented structures and situational logics in the English mental health system: theorising perspectives on mental distress in socio-historical context, Journal of Critical Realism.

Introduction

Understandings of the diverse lived experiences to which terms such as 'mental distress', 'mental illness' and 'mental disorder' are applied have long been highly contested. These debates, conflicts and struggles over meaning and practice are commonly characterised in terms of the different 'models of mental health', which typically range from biomedical[1] to psychological and social frameworks (Colombo et al, 2003; Davies and Bhugra, 2004; Tyrer, 2013; Davidson et al, 2016). The tensions associated with these divergent models have, however, sharpened over recent years. The controversy over the latest (fifth) iteration of the *Diagnostic and Statistical Manual of Mental Disorders* (DSM-5) (American Psychiatric Association, 2013), the 'bible' of so-called mental disorders, which was widely regarded as further embedding biomedical perspectives (Gornall, 2013), was followed by the intervention of Dainius Pūras, United Nations Special Rapporteur on the Right to Health. He called for a revolution in mental healthcare in terms of a shift from a biomedical to a social and human rights paradigm (United Nations Special Rapporteur on the Right to Health, 2017). Alongside these global controversies, debates in the United Kingdom (UK) have also intensified. Recent interventions include calls by survivors and allies for policy and services to shift from biomedical towards more social and social-justice-oriented perspectives (Beresford et al, 2016; Beresford, 2019), and an increased profile for trauma-informed approaches following the publication of the *Power Threat Meaning Framework* (Johnstone et al, 2018).[2]

This book offers a research-informed contribution to this arena of contestation. However, it does so not by proposing a new or refined categorisation of these divergent theoretical perspectives. Instead, it provides a contextually situated ethnographic exploration of the way in which the action environment of mental health services shapes and structures how practitioners, service users and carers articulate and utilise these different models of mental distress and associated practices within their everyday activities and interactions. This is necessary because, in the 'real-world' setting of mental health services, models are not just a scholarly concern but also inform particular forms of action such as care, support, treatment, detention and the deprivation of liberties. Therefore, while a focus on models at the conceptual level is necessary, I argue that it is not a sufficient condition for understanding whether or not and how particular models are articulated and enacted in specific settings such as Community Mental Health Teams. Moreover, and more importantly, the question of models-in-use has significant implications for how the lived experiences of service users are understood and how services and society respond.

The core argument of the book, then, is that the way mental health services are organised significantly shapes (although does not determine) the way practitioners and service users within this setting think and act. To put this another way, mental health services are action environments that offer either enablements to or constraints on the articulation of models (as ideational frameworks) and their enactment in the form of practices within such settings. Consequently, a satisfactory account of models must consider *both* the forms of knowledge *and* the situated contexts within which they may (or may not) manifest. The aim of the book, therefore, is to examine this interface between knowledge, practices and structural environments and understand the effects of their interaction and interplay.

Consideration of the latter brings into view the contemporary organisation and structuring of mental health services but also its historical context. Like the wider economy and other key institutions, since the late 20th century the health and social care sector, and mental health services within it, has undergone significant processes of market reform and neoliberalisation (Harris, 2003; Ferguson, 2008). As a result, there have been significant changes in the organisational structures of services through the creation of internal and external markets. These have fundamentally restructured the labour process of mental health work, with a shift from provider to purchaser (or care manager) in the 1990s and transitions from relational to informational practices shaped by target cultures as digital technologies became more firmly embedded, just over a decade later. Alongside these changes in professional practice, the roles of service users and carers have also been fundamentally reshaped, with individualised consumerism and personal responsibility positioned incongruously alongside longstanding orientations towards punitive risk management (Brown and Baker, 2012).

In this way, the book brings into dialogue two substantive areas of theory and practice that are usually considered in relative isolation from each other: models of mental distress[3] and neoliberal reform of mental health services. I will argue that this separation not only limits our understanding of these areas of concern but also, importantly, weakens our advocacy of improved mental health services through a partial analysis of the processes that generate and sustain current service arrangements and modes of understanding distress.

These dimensions of knowledge, practice and contexts of provision are brought together in the theoretical framework utilised in this book: Emergentist Marxism (EM).[4] This approach situates the various forms of knowledge (biomedical and social models and so on) as ideational/conceptual systems within the cultural domain, while the contexts of mental health service provision are a part of the structural domain and composed of organisational roles and relationships within wider socioeconomic systems. In their everyday practices, mental health workers and service users both shape but are also shaped by these structural and cultural 'emergent features' as they encounter and interact with them. These interactions between the structural and cultural features of the setting and human agency are, in turn, mediated by situational logics which generate directional tendencies for action within this setting (Creaven, 2000, 2007).

The implications of this for mental health services and their labour processes under neoliberalism are that institutional reconfigurations both create possibilities for, but also place limits on, the kinds of professional practice and associated conceptual lenses that can be offered, implemented and received in this context. As the book will demonstrate, by reshaping the 'situational logics' encountered, these socioeconomic and ideational reform processes create 'strategic directional tendencies' that narrow practitioners' and users' discretionary 'room for manoeuvre', both practically and conceptually, with significant resultant strains and tensions for those directly affected. However, as well as compliance, these logics and strategic tendencies also engender resistance.

The application of an EM approach thus enables a defensible explanation for the failure over several decades to translate a putative commitment towards more socially inclusive and psychosocial orientations in mainstream mental health policy and services into displacement of the longstanding pre-eminence of biomedical and custodial interventions. It does so by, on the one hand, identifying the role of market-based exigencies, for instance targets linked to revenue streams in National Health Service (NHS) quasi-markets, in reorienting mental health work towards informational tasks and thereby marginalising social-relational practices and perspectives. On the other, it identifies the deployment of psychotropic medication as a technology of defensive risk management in a context of the responsibilisation of practitioners, service users and NHS Trusts in healthcare markets. These emergent features align to form 'strategic directional tendencies' that reinforce biomedical and custodial practices and suppress social-relational forms of support. In this way, the book contributes to and moves forward the 'models debate' by examining the ontology of mental health services as a form of 'ecological niche' (Hacking, 2002), which is amenable to the articulation and enactment of certain models and practices while hostile to others, regardless of the particular intentions of policy makers, practitioners and service users (Parker et al, 1995). This assists our understanding of why some models endure while other newer frameworks have not taken hold within services in ways that might have been expected.

However, the EM approach also foregrounds questions of individual and collective agency. Discontent with currently dominant practices, ideas, logics and tendencies is also visible and this generates resistance. The book examines the countervailing practices that sometimes emerge to challenge these constraints in the form of micro-level social-relational and community-oriented interventions and nascent potentialities for wider sociopolitical alliances between practitioners and service users/survivors.

A number of factors from my own identity and experiences have formed a backdrop to my interest in this topic.[5] However, perhaps the most significant factor, at the point at which this research study began in 2007,[6] was my background as a social worker in statutory NHS mental health services and, for a number of years before then, a voluntary sector worker with learning disabled adults. My perspective has long been that a radical strand within social work provides a knowledge and value base from which the profession can draw in order to play a role in strengthening social and progressive responses to experiences of mental distress. This somewhat profession-centred lens for progressive change in services was further reinforced by many encounters with psychiatrist colleagues at that time, during which debates and (sometimes) disagreements regarding the role and utility of biomedical orientations were common. My tendency to perceive a straightforward social–medical binary among professionals was, however, unsettled by numerous practice and activist experiences, including engagements with social and critical perspectives and interventions developed by critical psychiatrists and psychologists (Bracken and Thomas, 2005; Smail, 2005; Double, 2006). Even more significantly, my increasing contact with activists and ideas from the disabled people's and survivor movements further destabilised my assumptions, in particular these movements' critiques of examples of social work's complicity with oppressive practices (Beresford, 2016; Ferguson et al, 2018).

Nonetheless, at the start of this study, my theoretical orientation continued to foreground key occupational groups and their knowledge bases as playing a primary role in promoting and preserving particular models of mental distress within the field. However, while this notion of the relationship between models and occupational affiliation persisted, it sat uneasily alongside my experiences of practising in teams with colleagues who did not conform to such simplistic stereotypes. Moreover, as the fieldwork progressed, I was further disabused of any lingering assumptions of the straightforward 'social worker = social model' type that remained. For instance, I noticed that practitioner participants from social work and nursing might challenge practices such as diagnosis at one moment and deploy biomedical categories and practices at another. Reflection on my observations increasingly suggested that how and when particular models were articulated bore significant relation to wider organisational processes and power relations. These dynamics formed part of the emerging problematic that the study has sought to address, that is, how to make sense of practitioners' oscillations between these different ideational positions and the wider structural processes underlying this phenomenon.

The story so far has been one of professional and personal experiences. However, a further identity has been important in shaping my orientation towards this research topic: that of political activist, in both trade union and other social movements, including the global anti-capitalist mobilisations of the early 21st century. These engagements reinforce my sense that collective forms of political agency have an important role to play in shaping and reshaping history and societal structures. This has relevance not only to the macro levels of economy, society and government but also to the meso level of the welfare state, determining the nature, forms and levels of mental health service provision, as well as to micro-level conceptions of the person (in relation to society) on which our ways of making sense of and responding to mental distress are founded.

Consequently, my political positioning in relation to this field of study is broadly located within what Cresswell and Spandler (2016) call the 'psychopolitical' strand of contemporary mental health movements. This position is 'Sedgwickian' in so far as, in the context of the neoliberal assault on the welfare state, it recognises the importance of potential shared interests between mental health workers and service users/survivors in better-funded, better-resourced and more democratically and inclusively organised mental health services, and a focus on the possibilities for mutual solidarities and campaigning alliances to achieve these aims (Cresswell and Spandler, 2009; Sedgwick, 2015; Moth and McKeown, 2016).[7] However, as Cresswell and Spandler (2012, 2016) note, these potentialities require significant attention to the nature and depth of political and relational engagements on the part of participants within such movements, in particular mental health workers and other allies.

Such political and ethical considerations are as inextricably bound together in my research practice as they are in my activist orientation. For, while the ethics of research always involve moral commitments to others, the nature of such judgements is complex and needs political contextualisation. I concur with Armbruster (2008), who argues that questions of the locus of ethics relate to evaluations of the locus of power: we negotiate preferential loyalties situated in our own moral and political convictions. Consequently, contra the neutral stance advocated in positivist science (Burawoy, 2008), ethical research practice involves taking sides. Lindisfarne (2008) urges the researcher to stand in solidarity with the social struggles of ordinary people, using the example of democratic psychiatry in Italy, where the 'negative worker' was enjoined by leading figure Franco Basaglia to stand against powerful institutions and on the side of the service user (Scheper Hughes, 1995).

Having outlined the background to my interest in this topic area and shared a little about my personal, professional and political identities and politico-normative orientation, I now provide a brief outline of the methodology of the study.[8] The project utilised an ethnographic method, with a first phase involving 12 months of participant observation, over a three-year period from 2009 to 2011,[9] during which I was located alongside practitioners within an NHS Community Mental Health Team (CMHT). A second phase of non-participant observation data collection took place in late 2018 and early 2019.[10] The value of such a longitudinal and long-term ethnographic approach is that it enabled me, as researcher, to get alongside and close to people, practice and organisational spaces over an extended period (Ferguson, 2016). It allowed me 'to swim with the fish', as Shah (2018) has evocatively described ethnographic practice.

The extended engagement alongside participants enabled by this approach has facilitated an in-depth account of the ethical and political contexts of user–practitioner interactions. This proved methodologically significant because it enabled me to observe, over the duration of the fieldwork, the presence then increasing absence of extended social-relational interactions between practitioners and service users (due to informational pressures). These absences had notable implications for modalities of practice, engendering (ethical) tensions and strains for and between workers and users. As Burawoy (1998, p 14) notes, 'institutions reveal much about themselves when under stress or in crisis, when they face the unexpected as well as the routine'. As a result of this emerging informational dynamic, the number and frequency of user–practitioner interactions at the CMHT declined, and my opportunities for such engagements inevitably became more restricted. Consequently, the 'fish' with whom I was able to swim were ever more likely to be CMHT practitioners rather than service users. This yielded analytic insights while, simultaneously, representing a limitation of the study. Nonetheless, I sought to meet with service users in the course of their interactions with CMHT workers as regularly as possible and, in addition, sought to understand users' experiences and perspectives through separate one-to-one meetings and interviews during the latter stages of the study. One further and final methodological point to note is that all names used in this book are pseudonyms, and a number of identifying details related to personal identities and events have been changed in order to preserve the anonymity of participants.[11]

Before offering an overview of the contents of the book, I briefly note some important context for the study. As I complete this text, we find ourselves almost one year into the COVID-19 pandemic and in the third national lockdown in the UK. This event has had profound effects, with escalating levels of mental distress within the wider population but even more so among existing users of secondary mental health services (Gilburt, 2020). For this group, the pandemic has further exacerbated existing mental health-related inequalities and intensified distress, with social (relational) distancing detrimentally impacting service users, particularly those with lived experiences of trauma (Taggart et al, 2021). In this context, user-led initiatives such as Mad Covid have played a crucial role in providing online spaces of mutual support for survivors (Mad Covid, no date). Meanwhile, for staff there have been tensions around the difficult balancing act between meeting service user needs and infection control measures, reduced contact with service users in many areas, concerns around the detrimental impacts of increased social isolation for service users and mixed views on the benefits of increased use of video and other technologies (Johnson et al, 2020).

Alongside the COVID-19 pandemic, 2020 also saw the growth of a global movement to challenge systemic racism. While COVID-19 starkly highlighted the impact of health inequalities for racialised communities[12] (Platt and Warwick, 2020), the Black Lives Matter movement that re-emerged following the murder of George Floyd by Minneapolis police, organised to contest not only police racism but also the deeply structurally embedded racialised inequalities and the collective trauma that arises from them, of which discrimination and violence by police are but two particularly brutal symptoms (Nazroo et al, 2020; Taggart et al, 2021). Data collection was concluded before both of these events, but while this means that the book is unable to address the impact of the COVID-19 pandemic for services, staff and users, reflections on issues of institutional racism in the mental health system are included in Chapter 4 and elsewhere.

In this final section, I provide a brief outline of the structure of the book, which is divided into three parts. Part I, *Sociohistorical contexts of policy and practice*, consists of one chapter. This provides a historical overview of forms of mental health policy and provision. It does so through an overview of four key phases, or 'conjunctural settlements', in the historical development of systems of mental health provision. This begins with the 19th-century asylum, moves on to the hospital treatment system of the early and then the community care approach of the late 20th century, before concluding with the current settlement of individualised neoliberal services. The last of these has a particular focus on three primary modalities of neoliberalisation within services: marketisation and performance management; consumerism and personal responsibility; and risk. Integrated within this chapter is an overview of a range of prominent explanatory frameworks in order to enable examination of the contested nature of understandings of mental distress.

Towards the end of this first chapter there is a brief outline of the EM theoretical positioning of the study. This approach is discussed in greater detail in Chapter 8. Readers who are particularly interested in critical realism and/or Marxism, or in how EM's lens has shaped the analysis presented in the fieldwork chapters, may wish to read Chapter 8 after reading Chapter 1 and then return to Chapter 2. For all other readers I would recommend following the order of the chapters as they appear in the book.

Part II, *Lived experiences of neoliberal reform*, is composed of six chapters. These present data and findings from the study. These illustrate a shift from relational towards informational practices arising from neoliberal reforms. They have significant implications for the forms of knowledge and modes of intervention utilised in mental health settings. Chapter 2 explores CMHT practitioners' experiences of these policy and practice reforms and how they have impacted on their ways of working. An exploration of the changes in organisational processes and experiences of support from the perspective of CMHT service users is then developed in Chapter 3. Chapters 4 and 5 present detailed case studies of two service users and the casework interventions they experienced during periods of mental health crisis that included in-patient admission. These chapters examine how their lived experiences were understood and responded to by CMHT workers, family and the service users themselves.

Following this, Chapter 6 presents findings from the second phase of data collection. This followed an organisational restructure involving the transition from CMHT to a new Rehabilitation and Recovery Team (RRT) model. This chapter explores practitioners' perspectives on the impacts of austerity, intensified informational demands and welfare reform. Part II concludes with Chapter 7. This is structured around in-depth reflections from two practitioners. The first explores trade union activity, nascent alliances and a (contingent) recent decline in levels of struggle, the last of these a critical precondition for the implementation of neoliberal organisational and policy transformations in this setting. The second highlights experiences of punitive senior managerial responses to informational performance in this new neoliberal organisational culture. The discussion includes some considerations on political agency in this context.

Part III, *Theorising knowledge and practice*, draws together findings and analysis with the theoretical framework for the study. Chapter 8 outlines the EM approach, which combines an account of (sedimented) structure, culture, agency and the situational logics and strategic directional tendencies through which these are mediated in the interaction order. On this basis, it is argued that mental health services should be understood as a 'layered' domain of co-existing sedimented and contemporaneous ideas and practices. These conceptual and organisational layers coalesce around strategic directional tendencies that reinforce biomedical and custodial approaches under neoliberalism. But resistance to these, in the form of countervailing ethico-political tendencies and social-relational orientations, is also visible. Mental health work should, therefore, be understood as a process involving navigation between these logics and directional tendencies according to the exigencies of context and the ethico-political positioning of the worker.

Chapter 9 explores, in greater detail, discontent with currently dominant strategic directional tendencies and forms of resistance to these. It also considers how these countervailing trends and resistance might inform the development of alternative social-relational approaches within mental health services. The conclusion then offers some final reflections on the political, policy and practice implications of this theoretical approach and the findings.

PART I

Sociohistorical contexts of policy and practice

Mental health services: from the asylum to neoliberal reform

This chapter provides historical and policy context for the fieldwork chapters that follow. It begins by arguing that models of mental distress cannot be understood in isolation from the activities and action environments of which they form a part. Therefore, to develop a more contextually situated account of these forms of knowledge, the chapter proposes a sociohistorical framework for understanding key phases in the development of policies and systems of mental health provision. These four phases, or 'conjunctural settlements', begin with the 19th-century asylum, followed by the biomedical hospital system, then community care in the 20th century, and finally contemporary neoliberal provision. Prominent ways of understanding and responding to mental distress associated with each settlement are introduced.

The relationship between knowledge and practice

As the introductory chapter noted, mental distress is conceptualised in a number of different ways. This has found expression in the diverse range of explanatory frameworks utilised by mental health practitioners, service users, carers and others to understand and define such experiences. The practice of mental health workers tends to be oriented by professional training and disciplinary background and this is apparent in relation to understandings of mental distress (Coppock and Hopton, 2000). The explanatory frameworks drawn on by the various occupational groups, service users and others in this field are commonly conceptualised as articulations of professional ideologies and knowledge bases (Abbott and Wallace, 1990). These encompass a broad range of positions, from biomedical models of illness and psychopathology, through psychological and psychosocial orientations, to social perspectives informed by sociological theory and recovery models underpinned by conceptions of service user empowerment (Anthony, 1993; Tew, 2005, 2011; Read and Dillon, 2013; Davidson et al, 2016).

Often, accounts of models of mental distress/illness within services and the academy abstract these forms of knowledge from the material conditions, historical processes and forms of agency through which they are produced, sustained or modified. This leads to an unsatisfactorily static and reified account of such concepts. Instead, I will argue that knowledge always arises from and is embedded in social practices and political contexts (Sayer, 1992). In order to apply this context-sensitive, sociopolitical and historical form of analysis to knowledge and practice within systems of mental health provision, I will propose a theoretical framework that combines Harris's (2008) notion of 'conjunctural welfare settlements' with Emergentist Marxism (EM) (Creaven, 2000).

A starting point for understanding conjunctural settlements is that systems of public welfare provision are shaped by prevailing socioeconomic and political conditions. The latter inform the kinds of welfare ideas and practices available during any epoch (or historical 'moment'). So the Victorian asylum developed as an outgrowth of, and was moulded by, the broader Poor Law workhouse system, while the mental health day centre presupposes forms of Keynesian welfare assistance to maintain income in the community (Sedgwick, 2015). Consequently each historical phase, or conjunctural settlement, is characterised by distinctive types of knowledge (models of mental distress) and forms of intervention (treatment approaches and therapeutic practices) that predominate during that era.

However, welfare systems are continually shaped and reshaped by socioeconomic changes and processes of sociopolitical struggle. These factors destabilise the longer-term reproduction of conjunctural settlements, generating ruptures which lead to the reform and sometimes transformation of systems of mental health provision (Creaven, 2000, 2007; Ferguson et al, 2002; Moth and Lavalette, 2019). Novel forms of knowledge and practice arise through these processes. However, while new conjunctural settlements emerge they do not fully erase preceding modes of thought and action. Traces of these endure, though adapted to new conditions. Certain features of earlier mental health systems thus persist within later settlements as repurposed 'sedimented' elements (Harris, 2008).

EM offers a framework for understanding these processes of reproduction and transformation of conjunctural settlements over time. The interplay of structure, culture and agency is at the core of EM's mode of analysis. Structure and culture are regarded as different kinds of emergent entity (or 'first-order emergent' feature) that pre-date the actions (agency) by which they are then subsequently reproduced or transformed (Creaven, 2000). In settings such as mental health systems, people encounter a multiplicity of structures (for instance, community teams or hospitals composed of sets of interrelated roles/ positions and material artefacts such as buildings and computers) and cultural forms (for example biomedical and social models of mental distress). They then sustain, modify or transform these structural and cultural forms through their activities either as an individual or as a member of collectives (such as mental health professions, trade unions or user movements).

Within the mental health system, these various cultural and structural emergent features (models, organisational practices and role relations) may be in a more or less mutually complementary or contradictory relation to each other.

Alignments between certain emergent features enable some forms of action, while conflicts and tensions between features may constrain others. People's roles and interests within the setting, in turn, shape how they individually and collectively evaluate and navigate these institutional dynamics. For example, while interdependencies and compatibilities between particular social and political collectives and interest groups (for example between the state and the psychiatric profession) may engender continuity and the reproduction of dominant ideas and practices (such as biomedical models), there are also contradictions and conflicts (for instance interprofessional, practitioner–user or worker–manager tensions) that have the potential to create ruptures leading to new forms of knowledge and activity (for example the promotion of social, relational, user-led and anti-oppressive approaches). These institutional and wider societal complementarities and contradictions, or 'situational logics' thus play an important role by generating 'strategic directional tendencies' that sustain organisational continuities but also 'countervailing tendencies' that propel transformations (Creaven, 2000). While this sociohistorical form of analysis is mainly implicit in the six fieldwork chapters to follow, Chapter 8 will outline and develop its implications in greater detail.

The remainder of this chapter will focus on applying the conjunctural settlement approach to the development of systems of mental health provision, enabling a more contextually situated understanding of models of mental distress and associated practices. Within this, prominent 'emergent features' (such as models of mental distress or organisational practices) that are associated with each conjunctural settlement and that remain relevant to, and sedimented within, contemporary mental health provision will be identified.

Conjunctural settlements in mental health: from the asylum to neoliberal reform

In this section I identify four conjunctural settlements in the mental health system in England. These are: the custodial system of the asylum; the biomedical treatment system of the hospital; community care within the Keynesian welfare state; and neoliberal service reconfigurations. Significant models for understanding mental distress and modes of intervention emergent from and associated with each settlement are noted. Moreover, although each conjunctural settlement represents a dominant orientation during its era, the discussion will also briefly acknowledge alternative and oppositional tendencies and forms of knowledge at each historical 'moment'.

The asylum system

The backdrop to the significant expansion of the *asylum system* during the mid-late 19th century was the advent of industrialisation. As a result of this socioeconomic transformation, industrial capital was able to exert a high degree of structural control over state policy levers (Creaven, 2000). Consequently, there was growing state intervention to generalise social discipline around wage labour through measures such as Poor Law reforms under the Amendment Act 1834. While this was predominantly focused on enforcing labour market participation by the poor, this also included provisions for so-called 'pauper lunatics' in the rapidly expanding, centralised and segregative public asylum system (Bartlett, 1999).[1]

The organisation of these new asylums was influenced by this wider context, with barrack-like regimes that paralleled the new sites of industrial production, the factory and mill, and the Poor Law institutions of the workhouse (O'Brien, 2000). Asylum architecture reflected this and, behind grand facades, the buildings modelled prisons both in terms of the concern with security and in the culture of their attendants. This custodial orientation was further legitimised by pervasive cultural associations between madness, 'danger' and violence that have remained prevalent since antiquity (Rosen, 1978), and which have been mobilised at various historical junctures to justify suppression and containment of those deemed mad (Pilgrim and McCranie, 2013).[2] As a consequence, in spite of the availability of an alternative therapeutic conception of 'moral' treatment developed in the previous century by the Quaker William Tuke, custodialism prevailed within asylum institutions (Busfield, 1986).

Furthermore, while medical practitioners had a prominent organisational role within this new asylum system, administrative authority ultimately resided with magistrates (Bartlett, 1999). This was a result of the significant countervailing status and authority of magistrates in the Poor Law system, but also of the treatment limitations of an underdeveloped psychiatric knowledge base, which was, by the late 19th century, strongly oriented towards eugenics (Pilgrim, 2008). Thus, magistrates asserted jurisdictional control while psychiatry adopted a subsidiary, primarily organisational, role managing one part of these wider punitive institutional arrangements (Busfield, 1986).

Consequently, there were two prominent first-order emergent features of the conjunctural settlement of the asylum. These were, at the level of ideas, a historically embedded *discourse of danger and violence* that was applied to pauper 'lunatics' and which legitimised, at the organisational level, a segregative intervention strategy based on *custodialism* (Scull, 1977).

The biomedical treatment system

The period from the late 19th century to the first half of the 20th century saw a significant growth in state intervention around social policy (Lavalette and Penketh, 2003). An important element of this was a challenge to the institutional containment strategy of the asylum. The opening of London's

Maudsley Hospital in 1915 marked the beginning of a period of significant expansion of psychiatric hospital and outpatient clinic provision (Coppock and Hopton, 2000). Soon after, the 1924–26 Royal Commission on Lunacy marginalised asylum doctors from its deliberations, but its recommendations represented both continuity and change for the asylum system. While promoting a new emphasis on medical care and cure, the Commission also legitimised the deprivation of liberty of those deemed mentally ill. These dimensions were carried forward into the Mental Treatment Act 1930, reinforcing both the role of the medical profession and the asylum alongside an emerging treatment rhetoric enacted via a range of somatic interventions such as paraldehyde, laxatives, chloral hydrate and later insulin coma, psychosurgery and electroconvulsive therapy (Rogers and Pilgrim, 2001).

This treatment orientation, the biomedical model, achieved a dominant position within mental health provision during the 20th century (Coppock and Hopton, 2000). The characteristics of this model include 'specific aetiology, a predictable course, manifestations described in terms of symptoms and signs, and a predictable outcome modified by specific treatments' (Pfeffer and Stein, 1998, p 1251). According to this perspective, psychopathology is determined by physiological processes (Davies and Bhugra, 2004), with mental disorders regarded as biologically based brain diseases (Deacon, 2013).

While the 1930s had heralded a transition in institutional practices and ideology towards this new biomedical orientation, the 1950s saw a more fundamental shift. The emergence of the 'chemical imbalance' theory of mental illness at this time (Valenstein, 1998) provided a rationale for the new neuroleptic medications, the so-called 'antipsychotic' treatments, such as haloperidol and chlorpromazine, that were then being developed and introduced (Healy, 2002). This period also saw a growing interest in theorisations of genetic causation,[3] drawing on studies of the incidence of schizophrenia in families (Kendler, 2015). These developments formed the backdrop to the 1957 *Report of the Royal Commission on the Law Relating to Mental Illness and Mental Deficiency* (the Percy Report) (Percy, 1957) and subsequent Mental Health Act 1959, which reinforced the conception of mental disorder as a form of illness that was amenable to biomedical treatment. Moreover, the Commission also institutionalised medical dominance in this policy arena by endorsing a pre-eminent role for psychiatry in identifying and diagnosing mental distress and removing remaining judicial constraints on psychiatric powers. This further entrenched a medical hierarchy with occupational groups such as mental health nurses (formerly attendants) subject to psychiatric authority. This hierarchical orientation also extended to doctor–patient relationships where considerations of patient autonomy were regarded as secondary to psychiatric evaluations of risk (Rogers and Pilgrim, 2001).

Thus, the two key emergent features of this period were the rise to prominence of the *biomedical model* of treatment, and the establishment of *medical dominance* within this sphere of policy and practice. However, while biomedically derived concepts and practices were in the ascendant during this period, the asylum system from the Victorian era, the context in which these were still predominantly enacted, was entering a period of crisis.

The community care system

In the post Second World War period, a new welfare consensus was emerging. This was the outcome of an uneasy alliance between state monopoly capital and the labour movement as their interests converged around the construction of the Keynesian welfare state (Creaven, 2000). This newly emergent system of welfare provision created a context in which new approaches to the community treatment of those deemed mentally ill became both acceptable and feasible (Busfield, 1986).

Hospitals for mental illness were reorganised to integrate with the new welfare state structure as part of the National Health Service (NHS). However, it was not until the 1962 Hospital Plan, announced by Minister of Health, Enoch Powell, in his earlier 'water towers' speech, that the move from asylums to community care began to take shape (Glasby and Tew, 2015).[4] Here the role of acute treatment in district general hospital units was to supersede care in the asylum, alongside new community provision. Additionally, two key provisions in the Mental Health Act 1959 further facilitated the development of community services: a requirement for outpatient follow-up of patients who had been discharged after detention; and a legislated role for social work (Lester and Glasby, 2010).

However, while the district general hospital units began to increase in number, this was not matched by an expansion of community care facilities (Rogers and Pilgrim, 2001). There was some increase in the provision of psychiatric services in primary care, but a lack of investment in residential facilities by local authorities because of their competing funding obligations prevented more extensive community provision (Busfield, 1986). Nonetheless, a new institutional network of community mental health service provision had emerged by the 1980s as the last of the asylums moved towards closure. These included, alongside district general hospital units, community residential facilities such as hostels, group and nursing homes, and NHS and social services-run mental health day hospitals and day centres (Rogers and Pilgrim, 2001). Associated with these developments was the emergence of multiprofessional community team structures (Bailey, 2012). These involved a much wider range of occupational groups, such as social work and clinical psychology.

A more prominent role for clinical psychology under community care enhanced the visibility of this profession's knowledge base. The prevalence of shellshock during the First World War, affecting middle-class officers as well as working-class soldiers, had undermined dominant biomedical notions of genetic inferiority at this time and led to greater emphasis on the role of the environment and a concomitant growth in the influence of psychodynamic and psychological ideas and treatments. But their reach was limited by the extent of their main setting, the sphere of private practice, which remained relatively peripheral within the United Kingdom (UK) (Busfield, 1986).

With the establishment of clinical psychology as part of the new NHS, and then the emergence of community care, psychological theories of causation – particularly psychodynamic, behavioural and cognitive models – became more prominent. The *psychodynamic model* is focused on the impact of early childhood experiences and attendant unconscious conflicts. Psychodynamic therapy is consequently oriented to the exploration of the meanings of current feelings and behaviours through past events to make latent conflict conscious and thus more effectively managed (Davies and Bhugra, 2004). The *behavioural model* emerged later and proposes that symptoms of neurosis are produced through maladaptive learning processes and sustained by positive or negative reinforcement. This approach advocates a process of relearning through behavioural therapy. The *cognitive model* emerged as a pragmatic adaption of the latter and is concerned with how elements of human reasoning and thinking processes impact on psychopathology. The subsequent cognitive behavioural model, which integrates elements of both cognitive and behavioural models, underpins the currently prominent cognitive behavioural therapeutic approach (CBT) (Davidson et al, 2016).

Like clinical psychology, the role for social work expanded within the community care system. While in the early phases of professional development, social workers drew heavily on psychological (in particular psychodynamic) models, this occupational group also brought an emphasis on social-scientific perspectives to an understanding of mental distress (Rogers and Pilgrim, 2001, pp 22–23). Two such theories were particularly influential. The first, social causation, proposes that mental distress is linked to social disadvantage and stress produced by class/socioeconomic inequalities and/or forms of discrimination/oppression arising from characteristics such as gender, ethnicity, 'race' and sexuality. Accordingly, mental distress should be understood less in terms of individual pathology and instead as a response to social determinants such as relative deprivation and injustice (Friedli, 2009; Wilkinson and Pickett, 2010; WHO and Calouste Gulbenkian Foundation, 2014). The second theory is social reaction (labelling), a sociological approach drawing attention to the way forms of so-called deviance such as mental distress are responded to and categorised, and how social roles such as that of the psychiatric patient are negotiated and maintained. Theorists identified with this approach include Goffman (1961) and Scheff (1984), who foregrounded the harmful effects of institutionalisation and labelling within mental health systems (Rogers and Pilgrim, 2014).

In this increasingly multidisciplinary context, approaches such as Engel's (1977) biopsychosocial model, which integrates biomedical, psychological and social dimensions, appeared to gain greater prominence within mental health services (Pritchard, 2006).[5] However, the apparent challenge posed by the biopsychosocial model to the biomedical model has not been realised, with the former more indicative of the pragmatic co-existence of a range of professional groups within a negotiated order in integrated teams rather than a genuine integrative orthodoxy (Pilgrim, 2002). Similarly, the challenge to the authority of psychiatry resulting from this expanding range of occupational groups under community care was contained by an enduring medical hierarchy within which professions such as nursing, social work and clinical psychology retained a subsidiary role (Busfield, 1986).

Nonetheless, other countervailing tendencies were apparent during this period. While the anti-psychiatry movement of the late 1960s initiated a popular critique of biomedical orthodoxy (Hopton, 2006), the service user/survivor[6] movement that emerged soon after with the formation of the Mental Patients' Union in the early 1970s represented the beginning of a more fundamental challenge to medical paternalism and dominant modes of knowledge production concerning madness and distress (Survivors History Group, 2011; Beresford, 2012). The user/survivor movement coalesced in the context of the political foment of the 1960s and 1970s, a period characterised by high levels of resistance to forms of racial, gender, disability and lesbian, gay, bisexual and transgender (LGBT) oppression as well as resurgent labour movement struggles (Crossley, 2006).

The movement drew attention to the long history of silencing and epistemic injustice (Fricker, 2010) that service users have faced as a result of oppressive psychiatric structures and treatment (Russo and Beresford, 2015; Daley et al, 2019). Service user movement activists were also instrumental in generating a growing literature documenting experiences of recovery that challenged the biomedical view that characterised severe mental distress as inevitably involving deterioration and chronicity (Deegan, 1988) and demanding participatory and user-led policy and provision (Beresford, 2016). Despite these challenges, dominant institutional structures remained intact. However, these struggles underpinned the emergence of some arenas of user-led provision and knowledge production (Beresford, 2016), alongside anti-oppressive, radical and democratising orientations within the mental health professions that have exerted an influence on some practitioners (Ferguson and Woodward, 2009; McKeown, 2020).

The systemic changes unfolding during the community care era generated two significant new emergent features. The first was an increasingly wide and eclectic range of *social-relational approaches* at the organisational level, including relationship-based casework, therapeutic interventions oriented to depth understandings (Luhrmann, 2001) and forms of community work. These were, in part, a product of the expanding array of community-based mental health professions during this period. Alongside this, social movements emerged to pose a challenge to extant power relations and inequalities within the welfare system and wider society. These social and labour movement interventions helped to engender the development of a second emergent feature at that time: an overt *ethico-political orientation*, which informed survivor movements but also influenced more radical forms of mental health professional practice, including anti-oppressive, participatory and structural approaches.

However, relationship-based approaches and multiprofessional structures are not *necessarily* a bulwark against individualised and pathologising models of practice. Meanwhile, radical and critical practices were predominantly limited to the margins of mainstream service provision (Ferguson, 2008). Consequently, mental health services under community care were characterised by both relational practices but also an enduring medical dominance and paternalism.

Neoliberal individualised system

The structural compromises underpinning Keynesian welfarism began to come under challenge following the global crisis that unfolded during the early 1970s. This was characterised by economic contraction and stagnation and marked the end of the long post-war boom. The response from significant sections of the state and corporate capital was to reorient public policy towards substantial reductions in levels of welfare state spending and a comprehensive programme of privatisation and economic restructuring (Ferguson et al, 2002). This, however, required disciplining of the trade union movement and, as a consequence, there were multiple labour–capital confrontations. As a result of the defeats experienced by the labour movement at this time, its organisational capacities were significantly reduced from the 1980s onwards (Creaven, 2000).

In this context, social-democratic perspectives in favour of state intervention in areas such as health and social care were superseded by neoliberal reform, which regarded the state's role as facilitating markets rather than direct service provision (Harvey, 2005). However, rather than constituting a static, singular blueprint, this form of market-led socioeconomic restructuring should be understood as neoliberalisation. This is a dynamic, complex and variegated set of processes, which are mediated by the contingencies of their particular institutional and organisational settings. These operate at various scales from the local to national and unfold unevenly over time (Brenner et al, 2010; Peck and Theodore, 2012).

This historical variability is visible in the shift from a vanguard round of neoliberalisation in the UK during the 1980s, characterised by aggressive privatisation and deregulation and, in the context of the NHS and social services, the creation of internal and external markets (Harris, 2003), to a second more technocratic-managerial phase of neoliberal policy reform in the late 1990s. This involved 'modernisation' agendas in health and social care, enacted via target cultures to further embed market norms (Worrall et al, 2010), and a shift from so-called passive welfare states to active 'workfare' regimes (Tickell and Peck, 2003). A third 'austerity' phase from 2009, initiated following the financial crisis of 2007–08, involved consolidation of earlier neoliberal reforms. This was achieved through cuts to health and social care provision, the ongoing erosion of welfare safety nets and increasingly punitive conditionalities to enforce 'workfare' (Friedli and Stearn, 2015; Theodore, 2019). These phases highlight the uneven and incremental nature of neoliberalisation (Brenner et al, 2010).

Building on this framework, this section will identify three core modalities of neoliberalisation in the mental health system and describe their overlapping and incremental development over time. These are: marketisation and performance management; consumerism and individual responsibility; and risk management.

Marketisation and performance management

Neoliberal reform has involved the creation of multiple 'routes to market', including privatisation, marketisation and outsourcing (Clarke, 2004), and this has been visible in the mental health sector and related social care provision. The NHS and Community Care Act 1990 marked the beginning of this process[7] by introducing a purchaser/provider split that facilitated the outsourcing of many health and social care functions in a mixed economy of care (Harris, 2003). As a result, third (voluntary) and private sector organisations began to compete in external markets for contracts to deliver services such as community and residential support for the statutory mental health sector. Consequently, staff from the third or private sector, frequently without professional qualifications, have become increasingly central to the delivery of services, carrying out non-core routine tasks that would have been provided previously by qualified workers from the mental health professions (Ramon, 2006, 2007).

Following the establishment of markets, neoliberal reform of health and social care services then proceeded through the introduction of managerialism via New Public Management (NPM) and target-driven 'modernisation'. NPM represents an important strategy for integrating the tenets of neoliberalism into the public sector by reconfiguring or dismantling public service bureaucracies. A significant initial step for NHS mental health services in this regard was the introduction, in the early 1990s, of a United States (US) influenced 'case management' approach known as the Care Programme Approach (CPA) (Lester and Glasby, 2010). NPM was further consolidated by the establishment of integrated mental health teams (Rogers and Pilgrim, 2001).[8] While the initial expansion of multiprofessional working was a product of the shift from hospital to community care, the neoliberal iteration of the integrated team enabled more effective and centralised managerial direction of professional practice at the organisational level. This restructuring of practice, in particular the increased genericism, standardisation and deskilling associated with the integrated team approach, has undermined the significant relationship between personal and professional identity (Onyett, 2003). This has been linked with reduced role clarity and role 'blurring' for practitioners, with detrimental consequences for morale and stress/burnout levels (Onyett et al, 1997; Evetts, 1999; O'Neill, 2015). Additionally, at the ideological level, these reforms have served to embed a performance management culture and inculcate business values (Clarke and Newman, 1997; Newman, 2007).

Subsequent reforms have further deepened the neoliberalisation of this sector. The introduction of NHS Foundation Trusts as service providers from 2003 was another critical juncture. Foundation Trusts function as corporate entities with independence from government control and are required to produce financial surpluses through competitive activity in healthcare markets (Pollock et al, 2003; Lister, 2008). A corollary of this market provider role is the necessity for mechanisms allowing the profitability of the various 'business units' within these healthcare organisations to be more visible and transparent (Monitor, 2006). The Mental Health Payments System (MHPS), formerly known as Payment by Results (PbR), which was introduced in 2013 to replace block contract funding, was designed to meet this requirement through increased commodification and standardisation of the products (that is, services) offered by Foundation Trusts and other providers (Pollock and Price, 2011). This was achieved through the development of a range of care pathways and tariffs based on the Health of the Nation Outcome Scale (HoNOS) 'clustering' system, which function as quantified and costed units of professional intervention commensurate with varying types and levels of mental health need. To facilitate this commodification process, Foundation Trusts embarked on a programme of organisational restructuring to reconfigure provision around service-line management (SLM) care pathways (this process will be described further in Chapter 6) (Foot et al, 2012).

The embedding of market mechanisms in NHS service procurement processes has led to a proliferation of monitoring arrangements.

Consequently, there have been escalating requirements for mental health practitioners to collect data and meet key performance indicators (KPIs) for a wide range of purposes, including the Monitor Compliance Framework, Commissioning for Quality and Innovation (CQUIN) payment framework goals, Local Authority Adult Social Care Performance Indicators and others. Performance measures in mental health services tend to align with managerial conceptions of efficiency and throughput, and orient summatively to supply and service content (Clarkson and Challis, 2002). This contrasts with the earlier Keynesian community care regime where professionals tended to have greater discretion, within the boundaries of their particular knowledge base, to define the goals (rather than measures) of their work (Harris and Unwin, 2009).

Data generation has thus become a central feature of the commodification of public services, and representations of performance a key modality for the evaluation of the effectiveness of organisations in competitive market environments. An important consequence of this 'informational' turn (Parton, 2008) is that the careful crafting of such representations has become a core organisational requirement. Ball (2003, p 224) refers to these as *fabrications*, which are 'versions of an organisation ... which does not exist – they are not "outside the truth" but neither do they render simply true or direct accounts – they are produced purposefully in order "to be accountable"'.

Fabrications, and the acts by which they are created (including institutional gaming), strengthen and reproduce the systems of information collection and management of which they are a part (Brown and Calnan, 2009). As a result, organisational purposes and the relationship between service providers and recipients have been reshaped. This has created tensions for workers in so far as various dimensions of professional practice are no longer deemed to 'fit' the presentational priorities of the performance regime. Practitioners consequently experience pressure to deprioritise established relational work modalities and ethical commitments and focus instead on the performative informational demands of institutional fabrication (Ball, 2003).

Consumerism and individual responsibility

An important corollary of the market-oriented restructuring of mental health services has been a discourse (and associated policy measures) that seek to facilitate, foster and promote consumerism among users of public services, as well as citizens more widely. This reflects a project aiming to reconstruct state–citizen relationships in ways that displace older categories of collective citizenship in relation to welfare provision and foreground instead the status and identity of *individualised* consumer (Clarke et al, 2007).

Central to this project has been the promotion by policy makers since the early 2000s of the concepts of user 'choice' and 'control' (DH, 2003). Choice has been constructed in highly consumerist terms (Hopton, 2006), with its mobilisation resting on 'the twin pillars of competition and plurality of provision' (Valsraj and Gardner, 2007, p 61). The previous section described the creation of healthcare markets to facilitate this direction of policy travel. However, this project was also dependent on a further 'pillar': a population of consumers with access to the requisite resources. The development of personalisation expedited this goal, utilising mechanisms such as individual budgets and direct payments to facilitate the planning and purchase of support packages by service users (Ridley and Jones, 2003).

But direct payments highlight some of the complexities involved in these debates. Direct payments are rooted in the philosophy of independent living and the social model of disability. They emerged in the context of demands from service user movements for greater self-determination, and reflect users' experiences of oppression and insensitivity to individual needs within the Keynesian welfare state (Spandler, 2004). However, these grievances were skilfully appropriated by neoliberal policy makers to articulate a 'rhetoric of producer versus consumer choice' and by NHS managerial elites to construct alliances with service user groups as part of a wider project to challenge the institutional power of medicine (Harris, 1999, p 921).

Other important developments such as service user involvement, self-management and the recovery model also illustrate the tensions between their social movement origins and integration into mainstream mental health policy and practice (Beresford, 2009; Rogers et al, 2009). These critical concepts/ practices emerged in the context of deinstitutionalisation, with 'recovery' particularly emblematic of the user-led critique of psychiatry. Recovery offered a subjective and existential orientation towards lived experiences of mental distress based on personal evaluations of self-management and growth as an alternative to the medical paternalism of objective or clinical perspectives (Roberts and Wolfson, 2004).

However, while it has now established a prominent position within UK mental health policy (DH, 2001), there is a tendency to apply such broad, multifaceted and highly flexible meanings to recovery that this concept is rendered potentially meaningless (Ramon et al, 2007). Rather than reflecting the transformative ethos formulated within survivor movements, concepts such as the 'recovery model', 'user involvement' and 'self-management' convey an orientation towards individual adaptation when operationalised within services. This is predicated on a particular discursive construction of the service user, as a 'responsible citizen' required to actively manage themselves in ways consonant with state-defined policy conditionalities and expert professional advice in order to minimise the consumption of, and dependency on, welfare state support (Brown and Baker, 2012). This orientation to adaptive self-management in neoliberal policy is underpinned by a philosophy of *psychocentrism* (Rimke and Brock, 2012).

This describes the prominence under neoliberalism of 'an outlook that all human problems are innate pathologies of the individual mind and/or body, with the individual held responsible for health and illness, success and failure' (Rimke and Brock, 2012, p 183). As the deployment of a notion of pathology suggests, biodeterminism is a core element of psychocentrism, with the aetiology of purported 'deficiencies' located at the individual level, in neurochemistry, psychological dispositions or personality traits, rather than arising from wider societal processes (Rimke, 2010). Furthermore, this approach notes how the diffusion of psychiatric and therapeutic discourses has accelerated in neoliberal societies, with the emergence of a concomitant culture of recovery underpinned by self-help. As a result, socioeconomic and political phenomena and their effects, for instance unemployment and associated stressors, are reconstructed as personal failures. Responsibility for intervention to address such experiences is thereby deflected away from structural intervention by the capitalist state and/or corporate institutions and devolved to the individual who is invited to engage in processes of self-treatment and social adaptation (Rimke and Brock, 2012).

In the specific case of mental health service users, psychocentrism invites acceptance of discourses of biological causation, while at the same time framing one's social and psychological condition in terms of personal responsibility. These elements combine to foreground the need for commitment to self-management through strategies such as adherence to prescribed medication.[9] This represents a paradoxical combination of biomedical determinism and personal voluntarism that, through its disavowal of the role of material and structural factors in the causation and management of mental distress, may reinforce the sense of moral culpability and personal failure experienced by service users if improvements are not realised (Dej, 2016). This is reinforced by the dominant neoliberal welfare rationality of 'responsible and active citizenship' noted earlier, which constructs the individual as blameworthy if these obligations are not met (McDonald, 2006).

In the arena of mental health services, a responsibilising and psychocentric orientation has been buttressed by developments such as the self-help philosophy of psychoeducation in recovery-based approaches (Winship, 2016). Thus, social approaches and forms of social-relational support associated with community care have been superseded by social inclusion imperatives to recover and to work (Spandler, 2007), which manifest in policy as an intensified focus on labour market engagement and the promotion of 'employment as a health outcome' (McKenna et al, 2019). These developments have increasingly delegitimised sick role status (institutionalised under the Keynesian community care system) and engendered distressing and stigmatising experiences of shame and self-blame among service users (Greener and Moth, 2020).

However, top-down initiatives and discursive interventions, such as those informed by psychocentrism, are contested and their outcomes uneven (Clarke et al, 2007). For instance, mainstream service user involvement approaches have been critiqued for functioning more as institutional 'technologies of legitimation' than heralding genuinely participatory and democratic transformations (Carr, 2007). Similarly, market-oriented policy agendas such as personalisation have been subject to critical scrutiny and challenge for facilitating the transfer of responsibility for health and social care from the state to the individual (Ferguson, 2007; Beresford, 2014). Meanwhile, the neoliberal policy appropriation of recovery as a means to de-emphasise service provision and foreground employment with the aim of reducing service consumption and purported welfare 'dependency' has also been challenged (Harper and Speed, 2012; McWade, 2016). The term 'neorecovery' has been coined to distinguish the currently dominant individualising and service-led derivative of this concept from its origins in grassroots survivor movements (Recovery in the Bin et al, 2019). Some sections of the survivor movement and allies have organised collectively against these psychocentric and consumerist policy directions, thereby highlighting the potential and actuality of resistance to such discursive formations (McKenna et al, 2019; Recovery in the Bin et al, 2019).

Risk management

A third modality of neoliberalisation is the rise of risk as an organising paradigm in public policy. Arguably, there has been a transition from need to risk as the central preoccupation of the welfare state under neoliberalism, with risk functioning as a core mechanism of assessment and resource allocation as the more universal forms of provision associated with Keynesian welfare came under attack (Kemshall, 2002; Foster, 2005). While there are divergent frameworks for understanding the relationship between risk and neoliberalism (for example, Beck, 1992; Rose, 1998b; Culpitt, 1999; Webb, 2006), the argument developed here is that the increasing prominence of the social production, distribution and management of risk within the contemporary welfare state is produced by increased demands for accountability in the context of market-oriented institutional reforms.

The following section will examine the implications of this within the mental health service setting. It will begin with longstanding historical constructions of danger and violence in relation to madness and distress, consider how these phenomena interact with novel and escalating demands for accountability and performance management within services, and argue that consequently mental health policy and practice have been reoriented towards actuarialism, prudentialism and responsibilisation.

It was noted earlier that stereotypes associating madness with danger and violence have a long history. However, such stigmatising constructions were rearticulated in the context of processes of deinstitutionalisation, which, although initiated in the 1960s, accelerated during the 1990s. In the midst of this transition, a series of homicides committed by people known to mental health services attracted significant public attention (Butler and Drakeford, 2003). In response to these incidents, a number of public inquiries were commissioned (for example, DHSS, 1988; Ritchie et al, 1994). While the inquiry reports frequently highlighted substantive policy concerns, such as inadequate levels of community provision and funding, the subsequent, high-profile public and political debates focused on the perceived link between violence and mental ill-health (Laurance, 2003). This discourse of danger was epitomised by inflammatory newspaper headlines, often with a racialised dimension (Butler and Drakeford, 2003).[10] Despite equivocal evidence of a link between mental distress and violence, this escalation of public anxieties contributed to popular support for increasingly coercive measures by the state (Taylor and Gunn, 1999; Pilgrim and Rogers, 2003).

This wider concern to manage the purported risks posed by mental health service users intersected with the expansion of market-oriented organisational accountability and performance measures in public services noted earlier (Lee et al, 2017; Warner et al, 2017). Consequently, policy and professional practice has reoriented towards *actuarialism*, the systematic collection and aggregation of risk data (Kemshall, 2011). This manifestation of the 'informational' turn involved a shift from clinical to actuarial methods in the form of audits, guidelines, protocols and tick-box risk pro-formas, reflecting an intensification of individual professional accountability for risk management (Rose, 1998a; Szmukler and Rose, 2013). Subsequent developments have been characterised as moving beyond a probabilistic actuarial approach and towards a more possibilistic *prudentialism*, where modes of risk management become focused on precautionary and pre-emptive constraints (Furedi, 2009; Pithouse et al, 2012). This was visible in controversial Mental Health Act reforms that proposed pre-emptive detention, increased spending on secure institutions and restrictive community treatment orders (Lester and Glasby, 2010). Community treatment orders represent an exemplar of this prudential approach, as evidenced by their higher than anticipated use (Weich et al, 2018), restrictions on user autonomy (Fistein et al, 2009) and challenges associated with securing discharge from them (Jobling, 2019). These developments have contributed to a prevailing organisational and policy atmosphere of 'coercion in the community' (Campbell and Davidson, 2009).

Among mental health workers, institutional responses to the inquiry reports and subsequent policy reforms have reinforced a sense that accountability and blame are being devolved downwards to individual practitioner level (Hewitt, 2008). This context of magnified media and legal scrutiny of individual decision making and responsibilisation has underpinned the emergence of an 'inquiry culture' of defensive practice (Muijen, 1996), thereby reinforcing these tendencies towards precautionary prudentialism, and demands for more formal procedures and training in the assessment and management of risk (Stanley and Manthorpe, 2001). This also manifests through increased monitoring of users' medication compliance to manage risky or challenging conduct, thereby reinforcing medicalisation (Bracken and Thomas, 2005; Foster, 2005).

Such pressures towards individual responsibilisation, as noted earlier, are also experienced by service users. The privatisation of financial risk has been intensified under neoliberal reform. This has meant that more universalist approaches to welfare predicated on an interventionist state and forms of collective solidarity have been weakened (Webb, 2006). Instead, financial and social responsibilities for care and support are increasingly transferred from the state to individual service users and their immediate social networks (for example, family), through market mechanisms such as personalisation (Ferguson, 2007). One consequence of this is to widen existing inequalities in this context, as the 'knowledge, articulacy, advocacy and assertiveness' of middle-class service users advantageously position them to access a disproportionate share of public goods within this marketised arena compared with those from more marginalised backgrounds (Clarke et al, 2007, p 107).

The earlier section on consumerism noted a growing emphasis on individual psychocentric strategies of user self-care, and this includes the management of risk factors pertaining to mental health. While there is a tendency towards less direct (supportive) intervention by the neoliberal state, the latter adopts a more indirect regulatory stance in the form of expectations of behavioural prudentialism (that is, 'responsible' conduct) by service users and this is reinforced through policy levers such as service or benefits conditionalities. In the case of mental health service users, psychocentric accounts of responsible conduct typically mean concordance with prescribed medications and interventions, and parsimonious use of services. However, the converse of this responsibilisation logic is that when conduct is deemed to have fallen short of these norms, the imposition of punitive sanctions is warranted. A rise in the numbers of people with mental distress incarcerated in prisons bears witness to this trend (Durcan, 2008; Brown and Baker, 2012).

However, these processes are not monolithic and uni-directional. The proposals for reform of the Mental Health Act first mooted in the late 1990s were met with considerable resistance, prompting the emergence in 1999 of a broad-based coalition, the Mental Health Alliance, to challenge this, encompassing survivor/service user networks, professional associations across psychiatry, psychology, nursing and social work, as well as trade unions.

This highlights the extent and breadth of the ethical and practical concerns concerning the harmful institutional consequences of the emergence of risk as an organising paradigm for mental health service provision. While ultimately unable to prevent the passing of this legislative reform, the Alliance highlighted the potentiality (although also challenges) for cross-sectional coalitions of resistance in this context (Pilgrim, 2007).

This section has highlighted three interdependent modalities of neoliberalisation in the contemporary mental health system. These are the market-oriented reconstruction of service delivery and performance indicator mechanisms, attempts to reposition service users as consumers in the context of the privatisation of risk, and coercive and responsibilising forms of risk management. Importantly, this illustrates the way in which the operation of power and domination under neoliberalism takes both centralised (for instance, state-driven reconfiguration of public services as markets) but also dispersed forms, that is, the (contested and incomplete) inculcation of consumerist or prudential behaviour in localised interactions (Sayer, 2012). The interaction of these three modalities has produced two main emergent features within the contemporary neoliberal mental health system. The first is the development of *informational practice systems* that have reoriented services and the labour process towards data collection for markets, performance regimes and risk management. These have increasingly marginalised the relational-therapeutic modes of intervention that formerly constituted the core of mental health professional work. The second key emergent feature is *individual responsibilisation*, which is generated at the ideational level by consumerism but is also an outcome of organisational restructuring around marketisation and risk management.

This chapter has developed a historical account of the dynamic and evolving relationship between ideas, practices and action environments as a basis for examining the complex and contested ways in which mental distress is understood and responded to in contemporary mental health services. The next six chapters will present fieldwork that explores these themes through the lived experiences of practitioners and service users.

PART II

Lived experiences of neoliberal reform

2

The transition from relational to informational practice

Part I offered an outline of the emergence of systems of mental health provision in England from the Victorian asylum to the neoliberal present in order to place prominent models for understanding and responding to mental distress in historical context. Part II presents an account of the fieldwork over six chapters. I begin in this chapter with an introduction to 'Southville' Community Mental Health Team (CMHT), a fictional name to protect anonymity. This includes an overview of the CMHT model, its structure and processes, and the range of mental health professions working within it. My main argument is that neoliberalism, market-based delivery and performance mechanisms have reshaped the labour process and forms of professional practice. Mental health work that was predominantly based on relationships has shifted to target-oriented, bureaucratic and informational forms of practice. This has generated tensions and stress for practitioners and service users alike.

Community Mental Health Teams: an overview

CMHTs were an important element of the closure of large psychiatric institutions and the transition towards 'care in the community'. Early forms of the CMHT involved both health and social services, although, at first, provision was uneven and fragmented (Langan, 1990; Onyett, 2003). However, the 1990s was a period of consolidation for the generic integrated, multidisciplinary CMHT model. By this point, it constituted the mainstay of community mental health provision for people of working age who met its criteria. CMHT provision tended to orient to those with so-called 'severe' – that is, longer-term and complex – levels of mental health need. But the 'balanced caseload' model meant that CMHTs also provided more short-term support to some people with moderate levels of distress. The case management model was the Care Programme Approach (CPA), which offered a form of individualised support known as 'care coordination' (Glasby and Tew, 2015). This model was contemporaneous and integrated with the market-oriented care management model.

From 1999 onwards, a range of more 'functionalised' community teams, including 'crisis resolution and home treatment', 'assertive outreach' and 'early intervention' services, were established to operate alongside CMHTs

(Burns, 2004). But the generic CMHT retained a central coordinating role. In this period, an array of key performance indicators (KPIs) and metrics linked to internal and external markets began to reshape organisational structures and professional practice.

In 2011, a further phase of neoliberal reform involved reconfiguration of this model to align with service-line management (SLM). SLM created new specialist clinical units providing services on the basis of particular diagnosis-related 'clusters' or categories of need (for example, psychosis, non-psychosis and organic) (Foot et al, 2012; Trevithick et al, 2015). While many of the functions of CMHTs were retained in these new units, typically known as Rehabilitation and Recovery Teams (RRTs), provision was limited to people with psychosis-related diagnostic labels. Until then, CMHTs had supported service users with other needs including those with 'non-psychotic' labels such as personality disorder or moderate to severe depression. Service users with these types of need are now supported in other service lines.[1] RRTs tend to have a more *formal* focus than CMHTs on outcomes and 'recovery', in particular managing the 'step down' of users to services with lower levels of support (and therefore cost), although arguably many practitioners already had such goals (Kalidindi et al, 2012). Southville CMHT was reorganised and reconstituted in the RRT format in late 2011, at the end of the first phase of fieldwork. I will describe this new model and practitioners' reflections on it in Chapter 6.

Finally, engagement with the hospital setting continues to feature prominently in the work of CMHTs, and now RRTs, even though (and perhaps because) inpatient bed numbers have fallen significantly. Inpatient mental health beds have dropped from around 70,000 in 1987 to under 22,000 by 2016. These bed reductions were initially driven by the policy shift from institutional to community care. But under austerity the pace intensified, with a 15 per cent cut in the total between 2012 and 2016 (Centre for Mental Health, 2017; Ewbank et al, 2017). Locally, the NHS Trust closed approximately a third of its inpatient beds between 2008 and 2018, a reduction from 365 to 235. But hospital admissions continued rising during this period, reflecting cost-containment pressures towards earlier discharge but also more frequent readmissions. Moreover, service users with higher levels of need, who may have remained in hospital during an earlier era, are now supported in the community, placing additional strain on service users and their informal carers, as well as workers in underfunded services (Glasby and Tew, 2015; NHS Benchmarking Network, 2016).

Southville Community Mental Health Team

Southville CMHT was located in a large urban centre in the south of England with relatively high levels of social deprivation. The CMHT served a local catchment area of 22,000 residents. The team had an ongoing total caseload of around 250–300 service users.

Southville was one of two CMHTs situated within a run-down two-storey, flat-roofed, 1970s health centre building in a quiet side-street near the city centre. The offices for the two CMHTs were on the first floor. At the top of the staircase, a swipe card enabled entry to the Southville office on the right. There were a number of rooms on either side of a central corridor: a rudimentary kitchen and toilets. Then two offices, one large, one small, housing most of the team. The manager, deputy manager and consultant psychiatrist had an office each. Team members based in the large office sat at one of four clusters of three desks that faced inwards towards each other, although with divider screens. Numerous pieces of paper were attached to the bright-yellow office door haphazardly with sticky tape and adhesive. One was a photocopied report from the local paper about cuts to mental health services, another the rota for on-call doctors, beside it a poster for a therapeutic gardening group. There was also a printout of a quote:

> We trained hard, but it seemed that every time we were beginning to form up into teams, we would be reorganised. I was to learn later in life that we tend to meet any new situation by reorganising, and a wonderful method it can be for creating the illusion of progress, while producing confusion, inefficiency, and demoralisation – Caius Petronius, AD 66.

Introducing team members at Southville CMHT

The staff team consisted of six community mental health nurses, six[2] social workers, an occupational therapist, a welfare rights worker and an administrator. There were two psychiatrists: a consultant and a specialty registrar (ST5), whose time was divided between the team and the local mental health in-patient centre. CMHTs also typically include a full-time or half-time clinical psychologist. But this position in the team remained vacant during the first phase of the fieldwork due to funding restrictions. In this section I will introduce team members who appear in this chapter. Names and some other minor details have been amended to disguise identities.

Evelyn was the team manager. An experienced community mental health nurse, she had trained in the 1970s. Evelyn worked first with people with learning disabilities and then moved into mental health nursing. Her practice was strongly informed by narrative therapy, and she co-facilitated 'My Story' workshops. Another nurse described Evelyn as an "old school manager".[3] Unusually for a team manager, she retained a small caseload, and her supportive and mentoring approach to her team contrasted with an emergent target-driven culture in the National Health Service (NHS). Evelyn was of White British ethnicity.

Dr James Bryant,[4] who was also from a White British background, tended to eschew some of the conventional markers of his status as a consultant psychiatrist. He typically wore black jeans and a dark-coloured shirt rather than the suit favoured by many psychiatrists, perhaps reflecting his penchant for rock music. The shelf above the desk in his office heaved with as many philosophy as psychiatry texts, and he once compared his practice role to that of the 'discourse analyst'. When we first met, he asked me if my study was political. When I said yes, he asked if I might like to attend a monthly gathering of consultants within the Trust with him. He explained that they, like him, would probably spend most of the time bemoaning their 'impotence' in the new NHS.

Filipe was a qualified social worker, an approved mental health professional (AMHP) and deputy manager of the team. He was originally from Spain and had an outgoing and gregarious manner. Filipe was enthusiastic about and supportive of the present study from our first meeting, saying that more social workers with PhDs were needed to raise the status of the profession in mental health. Before transferring into mental health, Filipe had volunteered and then worked in learning disability services, including for some time in a therapeutic community. This work, supporting service users to reintegrate into the community after long-term institutionalisation, was an important formative influence on him.

Constance was a social worker who qualified in the early 2000s and had recently completed her AMHP training. She had been with Southville CMHT for eight years and prior to that worked for many years at the voluntary sector organisation MIND as a mental health advocate. Following this, she studied social work as a mature student, a life-changing experience, because she felt the profession's values were congruent with her own ethical and religious commitments. She was of Black British ethnicity.

Southville CMHT had a distinctive identity for its practitioners, and for the way they were perceived within the NHS Trust. The team had a number of experienced practitioners who were mutually supportive, but also regarded as willing to be forthright and outspoken. "Bolshy" was how Kath put it, approvingly. Kath had qualified as a community mental health nurse in 1990, and worked at Southville since 1998, although she took five years out for maternity leave. Mental health nursing had grabbed her imagination while studying for her psychology degree, and she wrote her Goffman-inspired undergraduate dissertation on institutional interactions while working in a care home. But it also mattered to her that nursing offered a stable, reliable job and income. Kath was of White British ethnicity.

Welfare rights worker Martin, who worked across the two CMHTs, described Southville as a "caring" team, towards each other and service users.

This was important to him as he had initially trained as a mental health nurse but moved into advice work in the 1980s because he felt nursing then was too focused on the medical model and interventions such as electroconvulsive therapy (ECT). For Martin, who was of White British ethnicity, this caring atmosphere was, in part, assisted by the "laid-back and democratic" approach of psychiatrist James. However, he also acknowledged occasional significant tensions between James and other CMHT members.

Leslie had a similar perspective, describing James as "a conscious, caring" practitioner, willing to engage in "considered" positive risk-taking and thus unusually libertarian. Leslie trained as community mental health nurse while still in his teens during the 1980s. He followed in the footsteps of many others in his family by going into public services. He had worked continuously in the mental health field since then and, like Kath, had worked at Southville since the late 1990s. Leslie was a longstanding advocate of the 'hearing voices' movement and other radical and critical approaches within mental health nursing. However, when mentoring nursing students, he considered it important that they develop a good understanding of the biomedical model before engaging with alternatives. You had to "construct before you deconstruct," he once explained. Leslie was of White British ethnicity.

I will introduce other team members as they appear but will turn now to the labour process.

The labour process at Southville CMHT

Care coordination

A central role of all CMHT practitioners except psychiatrists is care coordination for service users under the CPA. The CPA is both the core framework for assessing, delivering and reviewing care and support, and the record of CPA meetings, which happen annually. Practitioners at Southville were care coordinators for around 20 service users, although this increased during the period of the study. Practitioners developed CPA care plans with their service users and did assessments and applications for social care funding. They helped with personalised plans and personal budgets. The role also included liaison with other services, most frequently the general practitioner (GP), outsourced community services and functionalised teams.

Care coordinators were required to ensure regular contact and meetings with those on their caseload. Contact was by telephone or face-to-face at the office or the service user's home. Practitioners retained a degree of discretion regarding the intensity and frequency of contact, which was usually managed according to perceived levels of relative stability or distress experienced by the service user.

Care coordination during 'stable' and 'crisis' phases

Team members tended to see service users as positioned on a continuum between one status commonly referred to by practitioners (and sometimes service users) as "stable" and another described in terms such as "relapse", "in crisis" or "acute".[5] When regarded as moving towards the latter, the role of services and mental health workers (and, increasingly, the service user and their carers) was to respond in ways that facilitated restoration of the former. During the first phase of fieldwork, CMHT care coordinators would typically meet service users whose mental health was considered 'stable' every two to four weeks, although sometimes less regularly. The consultant psychiatrist would often meet the service user only at an annual CPA care planning meeting.

However, care coordinators were also likely to have one to three service users 'in crisis' at any one time. Then, the care coordinator would increase the frequency of contact, and the consultant psychiatrist, the Crisis Team[6] or in-patient services often became involved. If the service user was admitted to an acute mental health inpatient unit, the care coordinator attended weekly 'ward round' meetings at the hospital, and worked on discharge planning, liaised with family and carers, and met the service user to provide support after discharge.

Profession-specific tasks

Care coordination was a generic task, and delivered by community mental health nurses (CMHNs), social workers and the occupational therapist. But team members also did much that was more profession specific. CMHNs administered 'depot' antipsychotic medication to some service users via injection. They also helped with the psychiatrist-led outpatient clinic, which was typically for service users whose mental health needs were regarded as below the threshold for CMHT allocation, or as follow-up support after discharge from care coordination. Several practitioners worked away from the office at the AMHP duty service on one day per week, carrying out statutory duties under the Mental Health Act 2007 (MHA), such as coordinating assessments and admissions. Although this had previously been designated to social workers, the AMHP role became generic from 2008. However, at Southville CMHT only social workers and the occupational therapist had trained to carry out these functions.

CMHT workers may also be qualified practitioners in psychological therapies. But the care coordinator role does not usually involve the formal and structured provision of therapy, although therapeutic skills are used informally in the course of casework interactions. Clinical psychologists, however, do provide structured therapy sessions for service users using approaches such as cognitive behavioural therapy (CBT), although at Southville CMHT the clinical psychology post remained unfilled during the first phase of the fieldwork.

Administrative tasks and ICT

At Southville CMHT there was also an increasingly prominent emphasis on interaction with information and communications technologies (ICTs) in order to complete bureaucratic administrative tasks linked to market logics. The beginning of the first phase of the fieldwork, in 2009, coincided with a significant period of transition within the NHS Trust (and more generally across NHS mental health services) from paper-based processes to electronic systems. This saw the introduction of the requirement for practitioners to keep records of contact on RiO, an NHS electronic care record system. Selected records were also kept on a parallel Social Services Department electronic database system. Increasingly these databases were used to provide the data required to monitor compliance with a wide range of nationally prescribed performance indicators and targets.

The most basic record-keeping task for team members was to enter progress notes onto the RiO system. These were brief descriptions of any face-to-face or telephone contact with service users, their carers or other involved services. The notes usually concluded with a brief summary or action plan. All teams across the Trust used this system, and so practitioners increasingly used it for up-to-date information on the service users on their caseload who were currently linked to other teams within the Trust such as in-patient, psychology or Crisis Resolution Teams.

There were several other important records. CPA care plans and risk assessments would be negotiated and agreed at the (usually) annual CPA meeting, completed by practitioners, then distributed to service users and other involved parties, and stored on the RiO system. These were regularly updated following any significant changes in the service user's circumstances. A further significant record of practice and decision making was contained within the letters written by team members. Typically, these would share information with a service user's GP, who retained an overall coordinating role for the health needs of their patient. These letters would usually relate to any service changes, for instance updating the GP when their patient was discharged from a service or ward. Practitioners might also write and receive letters of referral to and from other teams, often accompanied by standardised needs assessment forms.

Another major administrative task was social care needs assessment forms, which involved the collection and presentation of evidence for funding applications to meet needs relating to support around independent living, care, housing and social and community engagement. Social circumstances reports had to be filled out whenever a service user who had been admitted to hospital under the MHA appealed against their detention. Practitioners were also required to complete documentation related to specialist roles, for instance occupational therapy assessment tools, or to circumscribed functions such as AMHP duties.

This list is merely indicative and is certainly not comprehensive. In part this reflects the intensification of existing professional tasks. But a whole new array of targets linked to funding streams created additional administrative burdens for practitioners. A competitive managerial culture of continuous monitoring of these KPIs began to emerge with team performance measured using a traffic-light system. While these KPIs and associated informational practice systems created more pressure for practitioners, there is very little evidence they have improved quality or efficiency (Roland and Guthrie, 2016; Collins, 2019).

Market-oriented informational tasks were intruding into a sphere where human relationships had been dominant. Practitioners felt and often said that the additional burden placed on them by the production, collection and management of data reduced their contact time with service users and other professionals. It thereby eroded their capacity to engage in established relational modes of professional practice.

Impacts of neoliberalism on professional practice

In this section I present data from the study to elucidate the impacts of neoliberal organisational reforms on frontline practice at Southville CMHT. I begin with practitioners' perspectives on the implications for professional practice of meso-level reconfigurations of NHS mental health services, then the micro-level effects of the restructuring of mental health workers' labour process, the impact of neoliberal policy discourses on service delivery and finally practitioner responses and resistance to these organisational and policy changes.

Reconfiguring mental health provision

Organisational reconfigurations of NHS services driven by marketisation and managerialism had three distinct dimensions: outsourcing and competition; service restructuring; and new divisions of labour.

Outsourcing and competition

Community mental health nurse Leslie felt that there was a "significant difference" in the CMHT worker role compared with the 1990s when he first went into the nursing profession. This was due to the *outsourcing* of more direct support tasks to the third sector, and a concomitant reorienting of his role towards care management. These processes fed into concerns among practitioners about the implications of these reforms for the deprofessionalisation of CMHT worker roles (Ferguson, 2007; Bhugra, 2008). But people tended to speak of their disquiet in terms of the negative impacts on service delivery rather than professional status. For Leslie, a primary issue was that opportunities to engage in relationship-based therapeutic practice with service users and communities were diminishing.

Consultant psychiatrist James was worried about the lower skill level among third sector support staff and consequent quality of provision. He said this was a factor in the breakdown of a community hostel placement for a service user with complex needs. "It's harder for hostel staff than for us, you know. It's not like a ward, where they've got lots of trained staff, they're a hostel, so it is harder and they're not as trained ... they just can't cope with it."

Another emergent feature of this new landscape was the promotion of intra-organisational *competition*. Senior management at the NHS Trust built a competitive culture by introducing a traffic-light system to signal performance and enable comparisons between teams' levels of achieved outcomes on KPIs. They published these within the Trust to leverage performance improvements. This competitive atmosphere began to infuse the relationships between teams at the Trust, creating stress and anxiety among practitioners who wanted to avoid the ignominy of a poor placing in the KPI league table and the associated potential financial, disciplinary and reputational sanctions.

Service restructuring

Another way neoliberalism affected the team was recurrent organisational change. In its first 30 years, the NHS experienced just one major reorganisation. But during the neoliberal era, such reconfigurations have become an increasingly regular feature (Hyde et al, 2016).

During the fieldwork, only three years after the previous reorganisation within the Trust, the team was informed that there would be a major restructure of CMHTs to align with the requirements of SLM and its Mental Health Payments System/Payment by Results (MHPS/PbR) funding mechanisms. The market-oriented focus of this new model of provision was apparent at the SLM launch event. There Terry, an assistant director within the NHS Trust, explained that service lines constitute "business units", and that the Trust was seeking to gauge whether it was positioned "as a market leader" in this new competitive NHS service environment.

Many practitioners at Southville, such as Bill, were highly critical of these cyclical restructuring processes. Bill was a community mental health nurse, who trained in the late 1980s. He had worked his whole career in the local area, apart from a short career break in the 1990s to travel in Asia. He was also an avid cyclist and of White British ethnicity. Bill disapproved of the new culture of short-termism and incessant organisational change in the NHS, in particular because of its role in undermining attempts to sustain supportive and mutual structures and relationships within the team.

The restructure also raised the spectre of redundancies, and colleagues competing for a reduced number of posts. Anxiety became apparent in some practitioners' talk about how their skill set compared with that of others in the team, and whether this would be enough for them to keep their job. Abbie, the most recent recruit to the team, was particularly worried about whether her practice "toolbox", as she put it, would be sufficient. These demands had intensified significantly since she qualified as a mental health nurse in the early 1990s. During her school days, what had appealed to Abbie was that nursing seemed a "good, steady profession". Nonetheless, after 20 years based in a day hospital and then in in-patient settings she felt ready for the challenge at Southville, her first CMHT post. She felt she would have been "overwhelmed" by managing a community caseload if she had tried it earlier.

Offering a distinctive skill set was also a concern for Kerry, the team's only occupational therapist. Kerry, who was of White British ethnicity, had qualified in the early 1990s and since then worked mostly in mental health in-patient settings. She joined Southville CMHT six years ago, and had recently completed her AMHP training. Kerry said that as "an OT [occupational therapist] in the Trust we are having to get our act together and start using those tools to show to management this is what we can do … And please don't sack us".

Changing divisions of labour

A further trend, related to service reorganisation, was the restructuring of the division of labour within the team workforce. This had accelerated over recent years. Fragmentation, deskilling and specialisation within the labour process were driven by an overarching organisational impetus towards cost reduction. Chapter 1 highlighted the increasingly prominent array of targets and performance indicators, linked to funding streams for NHS Trusts and Social Services Departments, towards which professional practice and organisational systems are increasingly oriented. These mechanisms foreground the informational dimensions of practice.

Ruth said: "Maybe we spent a third of our time on paperwork years ago, but now we're spending at least half or more. If we were to do all the targets, we'd be probably spending two thirds of our time on paperwork." For Ruth, who had done a psychology degree and worked for years in mental health housing before training in social work, these bureaucratic demands were deeply frustrating. Ruth, who was from a White British background, commented, with bitter irony, that she was considering recording the following for her office voicemail message: "I can't get to the phone now or see patients because of my new role as data inputter for RiO."

Similarly, psychiatrist James described how the new RiO database system was taking him "one hour of admin for every hour of assessment". That hour involved 250 computer clicks instead of the 15 minutes of recording per hour's assessment before its introduction. This expanding emphasis on informational labour squeezed out the spaces for the more complex, indeterminate, relational and therapeutic elements of practice. Consequently, practitioners felt deskilled.

Deskilling also arose from increased specialisation in both the outpatient clinic work of psychiatrists and the role of clinical psychologists. CMHN Leslie explained that outpatients had once at least offered the potential for therapeutic engagement between psychiatrist and service user. But now the psychiatrist's "therapeutic skills, that set of talking skills, if you like, has been eroded. And increasingly outpatients are kind of psycho-pharmacology clinics."

James said that:

'In the 1960s and '70s, it's not that far back. But psychiatrists were the people who were doing a lot of the psychology, psychotherapists were mostly psychiatrists. But [now] psychological therapy is the domain of psychologists, and psychiatrists have become more, you know, biological ... So the definition of the role of the psychiatrist was limited to the, to psychopharmacology, to dishing drugs and that's never been what the role of the psychiatrist has been restricted to in the past ... But now our domain is medicines.'

The other key element in the restructuring of CMHT work was *labour substitution* through new 'skill mix' settlements (Mather and Seifert, 2017). This was happening within services across the Trust. Management recruited support workers and 'graduate mental health workers', a non-professional role on pay bands below nursing grades, to take on some of the less complex elements of professional work.[7] Social worker Farooq had started his own career in this way within the Trust. He came to the UK from Pakistan, and initially worked with the Southville team to collect data on a study of the British-Pakistani community's access to local mental health services. After the study, he decided to stay on to help implement the findings of the study, then trained in social work before returning to work with the team.

Nevertheless, Farooq regarded this approach as the replacement of "professional with cheap labour". Although Southville CMHT was comprised only of professionally qualified workers during the first phase of fieldwork, practitioners were aware that the imminent SLM restructure would involve more graduate workers in the team. They worried they would have to take on a more practice-distant managerial oversight role, becoming directly involved only in the event of a crisis. As Bill said at the end of a team meeting: "If nurses are just sitting on a computer all day then they don't need experience."

The effects of labour process restructuring on CMHT practice

The chapter now turns from perspectives on the effects of structural reforms at the meso level of organisations to their micro-level impacts within the labour process of CMHT workers. This section draws on Law and Mooney's model of 'strenuous welfarism' (2007) to identify four salient dimensions of reconfigured work practices in the CMHT.[8]

Transforming practitioners' tacit knowledge into codified forms subject to audit and control

As noted earlier, there was a significant escalation in the extent to which practitioners were subjected to various forms of appraisal, monitoring and audit of their activities against an array of targets and KPIs, with electronic KPI data dashboards made visible to practitioners on their computer workstations. Team members frequently experienced a disconnect between their own professional priorities and the measures on which the Trust evaluated their performance. In this transition, practitioners felt that data inputted onto the various databases, particularly those that triggered funding streams, were increasingly prioritised over face-to-face engagement with service users. Evelyn, the team manager, said that now the Trust only "value what is measurable rather than measuring what is valuable". CHMN Leslie felt like he was just "working for stats" rather than with people. "The process of recording the job has become the job."

Roger, who had been based in the locality of Southville for his entire nursing career of more than 30 years, agreed with Leslie, saying: "I have a relationship with the computer now, not with patients." Roger was of White British ethnicity and a militant trade union representative, well known within the Trust for his left-wing commitments having led industrial action against redundancies within the forerunner of the Trust in the early 1990s. However, he expressed frustration at the current paucity of action by his UNISON trade union branch over these new informational demands and their impact on workloads and professional practice in the CMHT.

Consultant psychiatrist James expressed similar concerns about informational reconfigurations, describing the intrusion of the computer into practitioner–service user interactions as resulting in "a weird triadic relationship". The new pre-eminence accorded to data management was starkly symbolised by the occasion when Southville CMHT workers were instructed to cancel all non-urgent contact with service users for two weeks in order to concentrate on inputting data following criticism by senior managers that prescribed targets had not been met. For Evelyn, this performance management culture was "drawing the lifeblood out of clinicians".

Flexible intensification of worker effort

The intensification of workloads was most starkly apparent in the increases in CMHT workers' caseload during the fieldwork period. Social worker Farooq's caseload rose from 20 to 25. He described it as:

> 'Pressure to meet targets and you just feel, "let's do this, then I'll have some free time and I will be constructive". You don't get to that stage. This week you get an email that next week is the deadline for carers' assessment so you kind of think OK. The following week you get an email that next month there will be an audit of CPA so you have to get all the CPAs up to date. Then another, something else, then it comes back to carers' assessments, or the information provided for carers' assessment is not complete. Or it's lost. It's just chaos.'

At one meeting, Alan, who was the UNISON trade union representative for Southville's social workers and based in another CMHT in the Trust, used the phrase "feed the beast" to describe these constant and insatiable organisational demands on practitioners to collect and input data. Moreover, Farooq said that the ICT systems introduced to facilitate this new set of informational demands were experienced as barely fit for purpose.

In order to facilitate these escalating and intensified requirements for data production, the work environment was spatially and temporally reconfigured. Practitioners previously had their own desks, but hot-desking was introduced. Manager Evelyn said it was "like a factory", with people squeezed together in rows. Senior managers also began to demand extensions to the temporal routines of the workers. At a managers' meeting, assistant director Derek criticised CMHTs' limited 'nine to five' opening hours. He compared this to having to settle for an 11am appointment with his GP that would mean his "working day is finished", as he urged greater flexibility.

Administrative burdens reduce time for care and support of service users

CMHN Leslie described how managerialist reconfiguration, work intensification and associated time pressures constrained the spaces for direct practice with service users:

'There's people in every community mental health team, social workers, CPNs [community psychiatric nurses] and OTs [occupational therapists], who've got lots of skills and abilities to offer people, who are not being allowed the opportunity to do it at the moment, because of the complexities of care coordination, bureaucracy, funding issues and so on that we're getting bogged down in.'

Ruth had chosen to work in mental health social work because, historically, there had been more space for face-to-face therapeutic work than other areas such as child protection. She bemoaned the significant reductions in contact time that now limited her opportunities for therapeutic interaction. Social worker Yvonne, who was of Black British ethnicity and had worked in the team for ten years, had to reduce the frequency of meetings with her service users from two-weekly to monthly. She lamented this, having initially been drawn to social work as a relationship-based career because of a formative experience caring for her grandmother as a child.

Constance described her fear that desk work was making her a "robot" rather than emotionally engaged. She was troubled by this, as she felt it conflicted with her personal and religious values. CMHN Roger used the same metaphor. He said he was determined to treat service users with warmth, not like "some sort of nurse robot". These anxieties and aspirations highlight the significance of emotional labour in mental health practice. The associated 'occupational hazard' of estrangement is sometimes a necessary defence mechanism against stress. But it can become toxic when chronically stressful working conditions produce more profound disengagement and burnout (Gregor, 2010).

Loss of breathing space and porous time

CMHN Kath described having "no time to think" in contemporary practice. She felt that Trusts no longer valued reflection, "as long as we fill the forms in". Social worker Ruth said:

'I can remember doing my social work training, reflective practitioner you know. What's a reflective practitioner [now]? We don't have time to reflect, we don't have time to think about how we're working with somebody or get new ideas. I mean in supervision there's a very limited amount of time because again supervision has become what our team meetings have become, which is all about targets.'

Practitioners coined spatial metaphors such as "corridor psychiatry" (the venue for the hurried conversation with the consultant) and "desk nursing" to describe these new constraints on practice as the outward gaze towards service users and the community became an inward gaze at a computer screen.

Responsibilisation in the CMHT: policy discourses of consumerism, recovery and risk

Chapter 1 described the intersecting discourses of consumerism, personalisation, recovery and risk, which have played an important ideational role in neoliberal reform agendas. This section examines how the principles underpinning these are embedded in mental health service provision and in 'responsibilising' service users and practitioners in a context of wider service retrenchment.

In mental health services, a major policy vehicle for consumerist discourses has been the personalisation agenda. However, these reforms have been found to increase bureaucratisation while deskilling practitioners without offering additional benefits to users (Slasberg et al, 2012). At Southville CMHT, practitioners described organisational pressure to promote personalisation options to service users. Some believed that applications for support services were more likely to be approved by the local funding panel if organised in this way. However, social worker Farooq was concerned about equity. He said that this new individualised approach had negative implications for some service users, because of associated plans to close collective forms of provision such as day centres. He argued that while some users were able to manage the new system of personal budgets, others were not, and likely to lose out as a result.

Several practitioners also criticised recovery approaches, in particular that implementation processes were driven by bureaucratic proceduralism and cost-cutting rather than user-led and person-centred values. These echoed debates, noted in Chapter 1, that neorecovery, a neoliberal appropriation of earlier service user movement-led conceptions, has been harnessed as a means to de-emphasise the provision of services and promote market-oriented responses to mental distress (Harper and Speed, 2012; McWade, 2016; O'Donnell and Shaw, 2016; Recovery in the Bin et al, 2019). For example, CMHN Leslie argued: "People have become focused on the stars on the charts, you know, the recovery star [outcomes measure] and the paperwork process, rather than the practical process of recovery and what exactly recovery means for different people, and the individuality of working with people".

CMHN and manager Evelyn talked about the housing problems of a service user on her caseload. Senior managers in the Trust and a supported housing provider had used the recovery model to justify a transition away from a more secure long-term tenancy model in social housing. Evelyn was angry about this shift from welfare universalism towards a more short-term conditional approach. She doubted whether the Trust directors would want to move home every two years themselves, as this new approach proposed. Kath noted that, as a result of such examples, practitioners now saw recovery as "a really weighted and discredited political term".

Personalisation and neorecovery have individualised risk and transferred responsibility from the state to service users. Meanwhile accountability for the management of risk has been devolved to CMHT practitioners whose work is increasingly refocused on behaviour monitoring and management rather than therapeutic and supportive interventions. Alongside this, re-emergent constructions of mental health service users as posing risks intersect with an intensified concern for institutional accountability. The result is an 'inquiry culture' of defensive practice in mental health services (Muijen, 1996).

One example is the community treatment order (CTO), a mechanism for supervised treatment post hospital discharge requiring service user adherence to specified conditions (Rugkåsa and Dawson, 2013). Southville practitioners tended to view CTOs critically or with ambivalence. Consultant psychiatrist James explained that while initially opposed to this "coercive" measure when it was introduced in 2008, he had now been "socialised into CTOs". However, Yvonne opposed and sometimes challenged these in her AMHP role. "They say it's a protective measure, but I think it's a way of getting people out of hospital a lot quicker." She felt these earlier discharges from in-patient wards were driven by funding cuts and bed reductions and facilitated by CTOs. "One particular consultant puts everyone on a CTO," she said. "I refuse."

Like Yvonne, Farooq was deeply concerned that CTOs were being signed off by psychiatrists to free up hospital beds. He also highlighted the effects of the institutional pressures on practitioners to align with defensive practices in relation to risk. For example, he received an MHA assessment referral on a Friday afternoon, right at the end of the working week. Farooq and the psychiatrists concerned assessed the male service user at short notice and then admitted him to the ward under section 3 of the MHA, even though none regarded this as fully warranted. Farooq felt highly conflicted, but both he and the psychiatrists felt they had to "cover [their] back".

The changing labour process at Southville CMHT: from relational to informational practice

The discussion so far has highlighted the extent to which the terrain of knowledge and practice on which mental health services operate is undergoing a significant shift away from a concern with the *relational* and towards the prioritisation of the *informational* (Howe, 1996; Parton, 2008). It is argued that this transition is an effect of the restructuring of the mental health team labour process, which is driven by the wider exigencies of the political economy of neoliberal capitalism within which this process is embedded, and from which it emerges (Garrett, 2005). This restructuring process involved, first, marketisation/New Public Management (NPM) in the 1990s, and then target-driven modernisation reforms in the first decade of the 2000s. Recent technological transformations of the labour process via digitalisation have offered a vehicle to further embed market-oriented policy reforms (Pickersgill, 2019). My contention is not that social-relational practices have disappeared because of these changes. Instead, they have been subordinated to other market and target-driven processes, as ICT facilitates the escalating neoliberalisation of working practices in this setting and across the economy (Moore et al, 2018).

Situational logics and directional tendencies in practice

As Chapter 1 noted, the emergent features of the neoliberal conjunctural settlement include structural elements such as informational practice systems and cultural/ideational elements such as individual responsibilisation. These co-exist with sedimented aspects of earlier settlements, including medical dominance, custodialism, biomedical models and social-relational approaches. As groups and individuals (for example, practitioners, service users and senior managers) interact within mental health services, they encounter an environment comprised of this multiplicity of newer and older emergent features. Where these clusters of emergent features are complementary, and therefore mutually reinforcing, they form what are known as 'situational logics' that generate 'directional tendencies' in practice (see Chapter 8 for a more detailed theoretical account of situational logics). These logics and their associated directional tendencies shape, although do not determine, the orientations, ideas and practices of mental health workers (Archer, 1995; Creaven, 2000; Mutch, 2020). The next section will consider Southville practitioners' experiences of two of these directional tendencies. The first is 'biomedical residualism'.

Directional tendency of biomedical residualism

As we have seen, some of the tendencies towards reductive, medicalised and defensive forms of intervention at Southville are a result of wider organisational and policy reforms. It was commonplace for practitioners' contacts with service users during a so-called 'stable' phase to be reduced to brief meetings focused primarily on assessing and managing risks to self and others. Evelyn expressed concern about the increasing ubiquity of this approach, which she described as "sleep, mood and meds" interventions. This describes a mode of defensive risk management in which practice is reduced to an ensemble of provision and prescription of psychotropic medication, brief engagement to monitor user medication compliance, and risk assessment via biological signs and symptoms. CMHN Kath described this type of 'inquisitorial' approach as "the business end". She continued: "I don't do therapeutic work anymore. I feel like it's the Spanish Inquisition. I don't have time. It's just asking [the service user] things and then I have to go." Similarly for social worker Constance: "It's all about meds and risk here," expressing concern that "we've become obsessed with risk." For CMHN Roger, this dynamic was driven by "arse covering" in a defensive inquiry culture. The job was becoming "social policing". And CMHN Bill considered escalating bureaucratic burdens and reduced contact with service users to be counterproductive even in their own terms, because "the best way of assessing risk is to be with people".

Such modes of practice are rarely actively chosen by practitioners. Rather, these practices are imposed by situational logics and the organisational tendencies they generate. These institutional pressures are produced by the intersection of NPM-related informational demands generating temporal constraints, the responsibilisation of service users in a context of limited resources, and escalating demands for practitioner accountability and risk prudentialism through surveillance of users' 'mental state' and medication compliance. The alignment of these emergent features of the organisational setting generated a situational logic that significantly reshaped the dominant forms of practice at Southville CMHT by squeezing out and marginalising the spaces for more holistic and person-centred approaches (Bracken and Thomas, 2005; Foster, 2005; Moncrieff, 2008).

Countervailing tendency of ethico-political professionalism

The predominant response to these developments was anger and fear, with some practitioners considering leaving the mental health professions. CMHN Leslie said to a group of colleagues that he had reached the point where he thought: "Fuck the mortgage and go and work in Tescos" supermarket. CMHN Kath laughed with the others at this, but whispered anxiously under her breath: "Fuck the mortgage?" In a tone of bitter irony, Bill added: "You'd have more contact with the public in Tescos."

But these institutional pressures and the tendencies towards biomedical residualism they generated also prompted ethico-political challenges from practitioners. Roger used the phrase "diagnosis human being" as an ironic rejection of these emergent tendencies towards biological reductionism and to express an alternative normative stance. In a similar vein, Constance argued that an over-emphasis on risk management has the effect of dehumanising the service user. This is also an effect of temporal constraints because, as Kath noted, "the more you spend time with people, the less you see them as illness and more as people".

These responses highlight a widely articulated theme from across the range of occupational groups represented in the CMHT – the aspiration to engage in relational-therapeutic and values-based forms of practice. Most team members disliked the shift in mental health practice from longer-term therapeutic and relationship-based work to informational practices and biomedical residualism. It placed their professional values in conflict with the managerialist organisation of the setting (Luhrmann, 2001; Leader, 2012). But the points where these managerial and professional processes are in tension have the potential to produce resistance and, consequently, recalcitrant modes of practice occasionally emerged (Fairbrother and Poynter, 2001). My focus here will be on two examples that reflect a countervailing tendency towards ethico-political professionalism.

The first was the bi-monthly 'My Story' narrative group co-facilitated by Evelyn, Leslie and other Trust workers alongside service user colleagues. Together, they sought to create spaces accessible to wider communities, thus challenging the constraints of individualised forms of provision and the restrictions of eligibility criteria. The delivery of these sessions was not a formal contractual obligation for the practitioners. Leslie explained that this work reflected his own and others' ethical commitment to provide inclusive and egalitarian spaces within NHS services that tended to be medically dominated. Leslie emphasised the importance of creating such alternative spaces, which reframe user–practitioner power relationships and challenge "the medical model and its one-size-fits-all" approach.

The second example was support for a campaign, involving a number of service users, against Trust plans to close the mental health 'Walk-In' centre at Southville. Unlike the services of the CMHT, which could only be accessed via referral or the locked door of the ward, the 'Walk-In' had an open-door policy to those experiencing mental distress in the locality. Evelyn described how the loss of this space seemed to represent a turning away from the community, a metaphorical and literal closing of the door to the surrounding environment and its residents. The Walk-In had mobilised collective and relational forms of engagement that are increasingly marginalised in a context of individualised and target-driven recovery approaches. Evelyn believed in the need to develop and extend service responses that drew on and valued "the wisdom of and in the community". As a service user, she said: "You are an expert of your own life. It's about connections and it's about communities."

Evelyn and Roger both supported this campaign by service users, reflecting an egalitarian ethos of partnership with service users and a commitment to universal and accessible service provision. Their support did not ultimately develop into full-scale horizontal cross-sectional campaigning alliances between workers and service users (McKeown et al, 2014; Sedgwick, 2015). But Evelyn and Roger were overtly critical of the management decision and actively supported the service users' challenge to the closure.

These two examples of a countervailing tendency of ethico-political professionalism do not reflect the mainstream of everyday practice in the team. Nor do they exhaust the articulations of recalcitrance and resistance observed in this setting. However, they do illustrate the ways in which some practitioners sought to create and sustain alternatives to the dominant reductive modes of practice imposed by neoliberal managerialist restructuring processes. Moreover, they indicate the potential to utilise the performative discretion intrinsic to these forms of welfare professionalism as a means to reclaim work based on person-centred, democratic and collective values.

Time, trust and relational practice

The previous chapter highlighted the changing labour process at Southville Community Mental Health Team (CMHT), in particular the shift from relational to informational practices. These changes are driven by neoliberal welfare state reforms to embed marketisation and consumerisation while promoting the devolution of responsibility for managing various forms of risk to individual service users and practitioners. In combination, these dynamics constrain spaces for mental health workers to engage in supportive social-relational interventions and reinforce defensive and controlling forms of practice. This chapter is about the implications of those changes for service users, in particular how reductions in time impact on the possibilities for trusting relationships between service users and workers in CMHTs. The chapter explores this theme by presenting the perspectives of six service users at Southville CMHT, with some additional reflections from their care coordinators.

Time, trust and relational practice in mental health services

The operation of mental health provision has long been characterised as oppressive by many service users (Crossley, 2006; Survivors History Group, 2011). But the advent of community care offered at least the potential for more humane and relational alternatives to institutionalisation and hospital care (Rogers and Pilgrim, 2001). Research evidence from both service user and service provider perspectives has identified the importance of effective relationships and working alliances between workers and service users. Within mental health services, the establishment of trust constitutes an important foundation for relationship building through open and cooperative communication and knowledge exchange (Kirsh and Tate, 2006; Brown and Calnan, 2012; Beresford, 2016). This requires attention to interpersonal, psychosocial and wider systemic levels.

Trust and relational practice

At the *interpersonal level*, personal qualities such as care and competence are key to building service users' trust in professionals (Calnan and Sandford, 2004). User movement critiques of paternalism within welfare services also advocate an orientation towards mutuality and the valuing of expertise by experience (Pilgrim et al, 2011; Beresford, 2016). Similarly, proponents of humane professionalism have highlighted how a collaborative dynamic can create a reciprocal and respectful exchange of knowledge and expertise (Pithouse et al, 2012). They argue, too, that orientation towards advocacy and holistic understandings of need help to build trusting relationships (Stewart et al, 2014).

However, to understand trust we also need an analysis that goes beyond the interpersonal to the *psychosocial level*. In particular, early infancy and childhood experiences of support by, and attachment to, caregivers have implications for all later relationships of trust (Pilgrim et al, 2011). Of specific relevance to mental health services is the evidence for the destabilising effects of the absence of stable early caregiving relationships. This can undermine the development of a basic sense of trust in the world, and of a secure and trustworthy sense of self, and lead to the existential condition of ontological insecurity (Laing, 1990). The significance of this psychobiographical dimension of experience is borne out by the very strong, although complexly mediated, association between negative childhood experiences and the development of various forms of mental distress (Layder, 1997; Read and Bentall, 2012). Breakdowns of trust in childhood have significant implications for the ways that people emotionally engage with, or disengage from, mental health services.

Contextual factors at the *systemic level* also play a fundamental role in either enabling or constraining the conditions for trusting, compassionate and egalitarian interactions (Spandler and Stickley, 2011). One feature of this is a tendency towards distrust of professionalism by the neoliberal state that is rooted in an analysis of purported 'producer group capture' of welfare provision by professionals (Law and Mooney, 2007). However, this section will focus on systemic changes as they impact directly on relationships between service users and practitioners. In this regard, neoliberal reconfiguration of the purposes and practices of the delivery of community mental health services described in earlier chapters is particularly apposite. In particular, the fragmentation of tasks and an emphasis on informational audit and risk management have undermined crucial conditions of possibility for trusting relational approaches.

This process has several interrelated elements. First, the informational turn weakens proximity, familiarity and trust between service users and practitioners. Second, calculative modes of risk management in services lead to forms of defensive professional practice. The experience of the instrumental and controlling dynamics of such practices further erodes trust (Warner, 2006; Brown et al, 2009). Third, the individualising neoliberal policy discourses of 'active', responsible citizenship and self-management go hand in hand with the demonisation of so-called user 'dependency'.

This is toxic for any conception of trusting and supportive user–professional relationships that extend beyond the short term (Brown and Baker, 2012).

These factors combine to inhibit the necessary conditions for atmospheres of trust within mental health services (Brown and Calnan, 2012). However, while the trusting and altruistic behaviour of mental health workers may be constrained and eroded by these contextual dynamics, aspirations to engage in practice oriented to person-centred, respectful and anti-discriminatory professional values nonetheless remain visible (Moth et al, 2018).

Temporalities of relational practice

An important factor shaping the possibilities for trusting relational interactions and spaces is that of time. This section will explore changing historical conceptions of time and temporality, and implications for mental healthcare.

With the historical emergence of capitalist social relations, labour power became a tradeable commodity. There was a transition from an earlier notion of time as cyclical and seasonal. Capital now conceived of time as an objective and universal metric to facilitate labour power's commodification. Profit was maximised by extending the working day or increasing the intensity of labour per unit of time. The process of embedding new rhythms of labour and associated temporal habits during the Victorian era was buttressed by the advent of standardised clock time. Earlier perceptions of time characterised by passing ebbs and flows were increasingly superseded by notions of time as a currency to be spent. New modes for disciplining workers included the dissemination and promotion of forms of moral disapprobation and the stigmatisation of non-productive or 'idle' time (Thompson, 1967). More recently, in the context of 20th- and 21st-century capitalism, a newer range of strategies has been developed with the aim of realising increased productivity and profit per temporal unit ('time–space compression'). These include the reconfiguration of production processes to increase work intensity through machine technologies, information and communication technologies (ICTs), labour process reordering such as Taylorism and Fordism, and just-in-time production modalities (Harvey, 1989; Wacjman, 2008).

For those categorised as 'mad' during the 19th century and thereby placed outside the labour market, confinement within the institutional spaces of the asylum was, as noted in Chapter 1, a common outcome. The temporal quality typically associated with madness and insanity in the asylum context tended to be one of permanence, an enduring and lifelong condition of disability and incurability. This temporal horizon endured into the early 20th century with the development of the diagnostic construct of schizophrenia and its associated prognosis of chronicity (Bister, 2018). Thus, the temporal *chronicity* associated with the asylum influenced the post-war emergence of 'chronic' as a particular classificatory term evoking stagnation in the form of constant and monotonous cycles of symptom repetition (von Peter, 2010).[1]

By the mid-20th century, the predominant emphasis within mental healthcare provision had shifted from custodialism in the asylum to biomedical treatment in the hospital. Modes of abstract, linear and standardised organisational time were predominant in this setting. This *clinical time* is associated with the routinised application of diagnostic procedures and tools, and implementation of evidence-based treatments (Hautamäki, 2018). However, in both clinic and community care settings of the late 20th century, more relational and therapeutic forms of intervention based on trust were also visible. These typically required the development of 'thick' relationships between practitioners and service users (Hardin, 1992). That involved a significant commitment of time by professionals to build up knowledge of, and exchange knowledge with, service users and thereby demonstrate care and competence in practice (Calnan and Brown, 2012). However, the more fluid and processual elements of this *social-relational time* tended to operate in tension not only with older conceptions of standardised, linear clinical time but also with the practical and temporal reconfigurations generated by the neoliberalisation of contemporary mental health services (Hautamäki, 2018). This emergent *informational time* of neoliberal mental health practice is underpinned by the technological reshaping of labour processes by ICTs. With technologies now inextricably embedded within the everyday practices of professionals, work intensification and 'time squeeze' are increasingly endemic (Hogarth et al, 2001). This underpins a broader lived experience for workers of a sense of relentless acceleration, time pressure and associated emotional strains (Wajcman, 2015).[2]

However, these informational reconfigurations of practice embed temporal reorderings of work in a further sense. An 'anticipatory' orientation invites and directs practitioners to refocus towards accountability at various scales by thinking about future consequences (Adams et al, 2009). Service users too are subject to this 'anticipatory' neoliberal time. They are urged to engage in practices of self-care and self-management and to comply with treatment and behavioural injunctions in the present as a precaution and protection against future 'illness' experiences (Alaszewski and Brown, 2016). This normative future-oriented temporality is integral to neorecovery (Recovery in the Bin et al, 2019). Notions of longer-term service use are associated with harmful dependency in this approach. Instead, neorecovery seeks to inculcate service user aspiration towards future-oriented goals, typically those involving timely efforts to achieve discharge and independence from services and (re)integration in the labour market (McWade, 2015).

The multiple and variegated temporalities just described are, it is important to recognise, neither mutually exclusive nor sequential. They are co-existent tendencies in mental health services. Moreover, this arena is characterised by dominant and countervailing temporalities that exist in a relationship of tension. For instance, informational temporalities are predominant in neoliberal services,[3] and these underpin the rhythmic ordering of labour for workers and the organisational tempos and time limits structuring interventions with users. But this is an uneven process, and sediments of earlier welfare settlements and professional practices nonetheless endure, requiring workers to engage in forms of synchronisation between temporalities (Cannizzo, 2018). However, there is also the potential for 'de-synchronisation' at the interfaces between temporal orders, particularly when these are in mutual tension, and this can lead to strain, stress and burnout for the interacting parties (Rosa, 2017).

A bottom-up orientation to countervailing temporalities can also be a form of resistance. This may manifest as assertions by service users of the complex and variable temporalities of recovery, articulated for instance in the notion of 'unrecovery' (Recovery in the Bin, 2019). This is a notion that the homogeneous, empty time of neoliberal performance management culture seeks to obscure. And there are also attempts by recalcitrant workers to practise in accordance with therapeutic rhythms oriented to the development and maintenance of trusting relationships over the longer term.

Service users' lived experiences of relational practice

This section will move from a discussion of theory to lived experiences. I present the perspectives of six service users at Southville CMHT. Service users are not a homogeneous group, and these summaries reflect divergent priorities and perspectives. But several core themes will emerge. The first concerns the nature, quality and purposes of relationships with CMHT workers, trust, time and power dynamics, dependence and independence. The second is understandings of mental distress and valued forms of support. Other prominent themes include historical experiences within mental health services, medication and treatment, risk management and coercion. All names given are pseudonyms and there have been some changes of particular details to preserve anonymity.

Val

Although there was an intercom panel at the entrance to the five-storey 1960s red-brick block of municipal flats where Val lived, the sturdy metal security door was frequently left open. Val's flat on the third floor was accessed via a low-ceilinged communal landing, well lit except for the occasional blown bulb. Val had given up her own flat when she inherited this former local authority flat upon her mother's death two years earlier.

While the brown and orange décor felt somewhat dated, it was clean and tidy, with thick carpets and numerous ornaments immaculately arranged around a compact living room. Val, a White British woman in her mid-50s, pointed in the direction of the bedroom where her deceased mum's belongings were piled up. She explained that she still desperately needed help to sort through them.

Val had experienced three admissions to psychiatric hospital. She felt the previous two could have been avoided with more support in the community, but the hospital "was probably my saving the last time". The time after losing her mother and moving house was a "dark period". Difficulties with transferring her benefits claim left her without money for an extended period. As a result, she barely managed to pay the bills or buy enough to eat or drink. "Finances were the thing that were making me the most ill."

However, on discharge from hospital, "only medication and not talking support or home visits" were offered by mental health services. For Val, this was a familiar pattern. She felt counselling would have been useful but, although referred, the third (voluntary) sector provider offering this service had too long a waiting list. Val was, however, receiving regular visits from community support workers employed by another third sector agency.[4] But she was frustrated with these arrangements. The ethos of such services was to encourage and support service users to develop self-management and independent living skills. Val thought that was inappropriate. "I'm deeply depressed," she explained, "I lack total motivation, so I really need someone to take the lead, and take charge of things."

Things came to a head when her support worker declined her request to sort through her mother's belongings under Val's supervision. Carrying out such tasks 'for' service users was considered to be in conflict with community support services' philosophy of self-help and individual responsibility to reduce 'dependency'. Consequently, Val felt that service users like her were perceived in negative terms. Service users are "not lazy and uncooperative," she argued, "but just take longer to motivate themselves". For Val, this revealed the extent to which these third sector agencies were not "geared up to mental health. All they do is come and chat to you." She thought workers should adopt a more practical approach. "They ought to be trained as more of a carer, and that would come with [more] understanding of illness." For Val, an illness framework was necessary so that workers were able to understand the limitations on her capabilities caused by her condition.

But Val felt she had been lucky with psychiatrists. "Mostly lucky," she qualified. For instance, Val thought Dr Bryant (James) could "understand my doubts and fears and how it relates in routine life". Val believed this came "down to [his] level of training and insight into mental health", which enabled a more comprehensive understanding of her experiences as illness. "A caring approach" was a second dimension of effective support she considered integral. For Val, the personal qualities of the practitioner, in particular "an empathy with the mental health patient", form an essential component of effective support. However, an exclusive focus on medication and a lack of personal empathy are too often the norm, she lamented. She said the frequent changes of support worker and CMHT care coordinator had been difficult. Her best experience had been when she had experienced stability with the same worker for "12 or 18 months".

While these relational elements were extremely important for Val, a further significant rationale for her engagement with statutory services was that they "can give medication and I'm deeply depressed and need anti-depressants". Considering her experiences through the lens of the category of "depression" had utility for her. But Val was deeply troubled when she found out by chance, on gathering paperwork for her benefits application, that she had been given a diagnosis of paranoid schizophrenia. That "made me feel isolated, that nobody would understand me from now on and I'd be viewed as an oddity. The diagnosis was never discussed with me. I didn't even find out about it until I came out of hospital." Val had doubts about the validity of this diagnosis in her case. "I don't hear voices. The diagnosis seems strange to me." On previous admissions, the only term psychiatrists used to describe her mental health condition had been "thought process disorder", a description she had been willing to accept. The schizophrenia diagnosis had come as a shock. She had "never shared" this diagnosis with anyone because there was a "definite stigma".

Kerry, Southville CMHT's occupational therapist, had begun working with Val after her referral to the team. Kerry's role was to do an initial assessment of risk and ascertain whether CMHT involvement with Val was appropriate and, if so, whether this would be short term or ongoing. For Kerry: "The trauma of her admission and then being in hospital and then being discharged actually made her quite depressed. My impression was that she'd been let down by services and you know, had certain things written about her that she disagreed with, and she hadn't really been listened to."

After her initial meeting with Val, Kerry had felt that the priorities were "listening to her, trying to reassure her and then trying to act as a go-between" with the third sector workers. Kerry also wanted to utilise a specialist and "very client-centred" occupational therapy assessment tool, as she felt Val had become "stuck doing very little. She was just tending to stay in the house and watch TV." Kerry thought that, "on the face of it", Val was able to just about manage. But she "could easily get lost, actually, because her risks are probably quite low. So, obviously until she really becomes unwell, I could see her kind of falling through a gap."

Kerry considered practical help to be both a means of building rapport and a medium of recovery itself. So she offered to help Val pack her mother's items, explaining:

> "'I can do that you know, I can help you.' She was like: "Oh no, no, no, I don't expect you to do it, I don't expect you to help me physically move and pack stuff up and you know." And I was like: "Well I can do." And she goes: "Oh no, no, no, you don't, that's not your role.""

Kerry understood Val's reluctance in terms of previous traumatic experiences. "She'd just been discharged and, and with Val you have to build that relationship you know, it takes a long time 'cause I think she was a bit kind of wary and a bit suspect as to what I could do for her, that's the impression I got." But Kerry could not find the necessary time to do so due to her large CMHT caseload and "all the other admin work that had got in the way". These pressures were a destabilising factor that reinforced Val's low expectations of services, and thereby undermined the conditions for the emergence of trust. Kerry explained:

> 'Unfortunately, there were a few times when I couldn't get there or I was late. And that kind of registered with [Val] 'cause it was like, it was something that she expected to happen, which is unfortunate. So I think to establish that trust and to actually get to the bottom of what was actually going on for her, it would have taken a long time, which I didn't have. It was very unsatisfactory for me 'cause I wasn't able to do what I wanted to do and I just didn't have the time and it was just a bit of a nightmare really.'

However, Kerry knew that Val was viewed as low risk, and in cases like that, preventive approaches were increasingly deprioritised at the CMHT. Informational demands and short-term neorecovery-focused community support were eclipsing the longer-term relationship-based approach preferred by both Kerry and Val. "The way we're going to be working, we won't be doing that [relationship-based] work," Kerry said.

Jorge

Jorge had a flat in an innovatively designed council block, notable for its striking triangular concrete buttresses that rose dramatically up from the street below. Inside the building, the door to Jorge's flat was located at the side of a large, and rather dimly lit, austere concrete walled central atrium. Once inside though, Jorge's living room felt like a conservatory, with bright sunshine pouring in through sloping windows rising above part of the room.

However, the room was sparsely furnished with only a sofa bed, an old television and a dining table on which, neatly arranged, were a copy of *The Times*, a Jehovah's Witness magazine, some letters and a packet of tobacco.

Jorge was a neatly dressed man with greying hair and a short, carefully trimmed beard. He had a strong Portuguese accent and spoke slowly in a nasal, monotone drawl, with little inflection in his voice or change in his expression. On a home visit I attended with his care coordinator, Leslie, Jorge gestured for us to take a seat at the table, and explained that he could not offer us a hot drink as he only had one mug. He then switched off his television, mentioning that he only really liked the politics programmes. Jorge was in his mid-60s and had moved to the UK from Portugal, via Spain and France, more than 30 years ago.

Jorge had been a service user of the CMHT for ten years, he explained, but he had been diagnosed with schizophrenia by his GP 15 years before that. There was a pause. "Whether I am or not is another question," Jorge said. Jorge revealed that he had had only one admission during those years, to the local psychiatric in-patient unit ten years ago. He found that helpful only in the sense that it gave him what he described as "the courage to survive". He then qualified this: "I didn't feel I had any difficulties."

Although he rejected the diagnosis he had been given, Jorge initially spoke more positively about the antipsychotic medication. "I feel more relaxed on it," he explained, "more relaxed and peaceful." But he quickly signalled greater ambivalence, describing little change since beginning this treatment. "I won't know how to justify not taking it to the doctor, so I take it." This sense of resignation was palpable in his next comment, which hinted further at the asymmetrical power relations within which treatment decisions were reached. "I cooperate with the doctors." The reason for his ambivalent stance became clearer when he described developing a speech impediment. He said it was because of the medication.

While Jorge was care coordinated by CMHN Leslie, like Val his most frequent contact with services was a community support worker who visited weekly. Jorge felt there was little benefit in this support. "They ask me if I need any help with cooking," he explained. "I don't know how to cook." Instead, Jorge preferred to buy a sandwich each day from any one of the many cheap cafés nearby. However, he had recently found the team's help more useful when dealing with a demand from the council for repayment of thousands of pounds of overpaid council tax benefit. "I didn't know anything about it, the limit" on savings in order to be eligible. Jorge stopped the story for a moment as he broke into a wheezy smoker's cough. He composed himself again, then described the outcome of the story. He had been required to transfer the remainder of his savings to the council.

Although Jorge was initially hesitant to disclose the experiences that led to mental health service involvement, he later revealed the impact of 'the

Force' in his life. "All hospitals have got the Force. It comes from Portugal. It's painful. There are voices and then it will stop talking, day and night, even when I'm asleep. It's bad." He continued in a matter-of-fact way, with no change in the intonation of his voice.

> 'The Force just talks to me. It started 25 years ago. I don't understand it. I used to have it as a child but it was silent. It causes problems, going to the toilet all the time. I want it to go off, leave me alone, but it won't do it. I keep it to myself. If you explain this Force to people, they'll think you're mad.'

Jorge described how The Force made him "feel like a prisoner. It squeezes my head." But he did not see it as an illness. He paused to cough loudly again. "I can't be bothered anymore, I just soldier on."

In describing his work with Jorge, Leslie talked of the need to work alongside people in a collaborative way to explore the meaning of difficult personal experiences such as The Force. Leslie tried to formulate responses that reinforce personal strengths and effective coping strategies already developed. As part of this, Leslie had brought in the Maastricht Hearing Voices Interview, an assessment tool associated with the grassroots user-led 'hearing voices' movement. He explained to me that this approach involved:

> 'Looking at the history of the voices, the nature of the voices, the origin perhaps of the voices, the coping strategies, the types of moods and emotions that the voices may reflect, the ways that Jorge has been managing them. And I guess integrating the voices within his life and managing and coping with them. And we tried to do the formulation together as well. I think that was quite helpful, just to have his experiences and not to get lost in healthcare or technical jargon.'

While not completely rejecting medication interventions, Leslie's approach oriented towards a focus on exploring users' personal experiences, subjective meanings and supporting self-advocacy and away from biomedical discourses focused solely on controlling symptoms (for example, see Dillon et al, 2013). However Leslie explained that, over recent months, he had limited opportunities to do work of this nature. He argued that, for Jorge, "who's quite suspicious and paranoid, being able to form quite a meaningful, trusting relationship with him was probably the most essential component of support and care for him and I haven't had as much time as I would like to do that".

Like Kerry, Leslie highlighted significant institutional constraints on relational processes and interactions with users, identifying three in particular. The first was the escalating "demands for statistics and paperwork". Second, the limited time available for work with Jorge was spent "being quite business-like". That meant, he clarified, "helping him with more practical issues, correspondence and benefits and so on", meaning less time for more in-depth therapeutic support. A third constraint related to community support worker involvement. Leslie described his role in "encouraging" and scaffolding the work of one support worker, who had formed "a quite meaningful and trusting and therapeutic rapport with Jorge". However, new commissioning priorities foregrounded 'stepped care' models of community support that claimed to reduce dependency and were thereby deemed more cost-effective (Joint Commissioning Panel for Mental Health, 2013). Consequently, community support services and supported housing providers working with CMHT service users increasingly offered time-limited provision – usually for two years. As a result, the support worker had to end his involvement with Jorge, and a new worker from another agency was brought in. Unfortunately, Leslie explained, the new worker and Jorge were struggling to build a positive relationship.

There were widespread concerns among team members about this short-term 'stepped care' approach. Leslie argued that, while "there's a place for it, you know, in enabling people to go back into independent living eventually and some people do very well at it, it seems almost like there's a one-size-fits-all approach at times". Furthermore, he bemoaned the way that these short-term models created disruption and instabilities that undermined relationship building. Service users:

> 'Are being shunted around, making a relationship here, making [a] new relationship there. Ok, you've done that, let's move you on here, let's put you there, let's introduce this worker and let's take away that worker because the two years are up … Why not give people a home, proper home, help them to put roots down, make connections within the local community, isn't that what recovery is really?'

For Leslie, these policy and organisational reconfigurations resulted in reductive forms of intervention that failed to recognise "the diversity of human experience, and individuals, and how they present". As a result, paradoxically, the mainstream neorecovery agenda undermined the potential for the kind of person-centred outcomes articulated in this policy framework.

Leon

Leon had recently moved into a 'supported living' project, similar to the 'stepped care' housing setting described by Leslie in the previous section. In formal terms, this was a registered care home setting, offering accommodation and support to 18 women and men with mental health needs. The project was based in a slightly run-down Georgian terrace overlooking a small square enclosed by iron railings. It is still easy to imagine this location during its 19th-century heyday, bustling with upper-middle-class residents. However, the council's present struggle to regenerate the area and reclaim this spot from alcohol users and drug dealers is symbolised by the installation of a playground in the square.

Turning back towards the house, I rang the buzzer to gain entry to the building. Paula, Leon's key worker at the project, opened the door to me. She led me through the building, past the staff office where three people were seated at desks, explaining as we went that she had been working on Leon's key plan with him earlier that day. We then turned a corner into a small meeting room where Leon was already waiting. The room had six chairs arranged along three walls, with large windows overlooking a small, sparse courtyard area on the fourth. In one corner of the room was a computer on a small table with a stack of dog-eared magazines piled untidily underneath, in another a large water cooler. Leon was neatly dressed in bright white trainers, light chinos and a grey t-shirt. He nodded a greeting as I entered, then looked down towards the floor again. Leon is Black British, of Jamaican heritage and looks young for his 36 years.

Leon had been with Southville CMHT for 18 months since returning from Jamaica. He first began to have unusual experiences 15 years before at around the age of 19. He had just started college where he was studying fashion and design. But one day, Leon told his mother, with whom he was then living, that he had lost confidence. And he had "started to have a few episodes", beginning to hear voices. As a result, he found it increasingly hard to concentrate. He withdrew from contact with his family and barely ate or slept.

I asked Leon what he saw as the reasons for these changes in his life. He paused and then in characteristically diffident and soft-spoken manner he said: "It just suddenly started." He explained that alcohol, drugs and "past experiences" may have contributed. "I used to take drugs, cannabis could have triggered it." After an initial period in hospital, Leon's family urged him to go to Jamaica and stay with his grandmother. He went and stayed for six years. While there, he explained, his uncle had urged him to try some "alternative medicine", such as traditional herbal remedies and baths as well as accessing Western medical treatments through a psychiatric hospital. Leon returned to the UK two years ago.

Leon described feeling better since taking medication. "I don't hear voices, the paranoia has gone away." However, he expressed concern about side effects, in particular weight gain, and was keen to reduce his medication dosage. Leon said that he also found talking to staff at the project helpful. Although he had not long moved into this project, he was already on track to move on to a self-contained flat and was looking forward to this prospect. With the assistance of his social worker, Farooq, Leon had also applied for a degree course in fashion and design and hoped to gain a place.

I was introduced to Leon's mother, Marsha, on a couple of occasions by Farooq. Marsha had worked for many years as a nurse. She recounted the story of when she first noticed Leon's unusual behaviours. He would cover the television when it was on and tell her not to speak too loudly in case they were overheard. Then Leon rapidly deteriorated and barely slept for weeks. Things reached crisis point when she arrived home from work one day to find Leon collapsed on the sofa, dribbling from the mouth. As Marsha recalled this moment, she brushed away a tear rolling down her cheek.

She called an ambulance and Leon was rushed to hospital. She explained how Leon was given a schizophrenia diagnosis, although she stressed there was no family history of this condition on either side. She had encouraged him to take his medication even though she was concerned about weight gain and that "the medication makes him sleepy". However, Leon tended to "stop taking his tablets when well" and she felt this had been a factor in his "relapses".

Reflecting on the reasons for Leon's experiences, Marsha identified his use of drugs. But she also mentioned that his father had died when Leon was 13 years old. A concern for Marsha had been that, since developing these difficulties, Leon rarely left the family home. Moreover, his elder sister tended to "do everything for him. It's not good for him or us." Social worker Farooq had then suggested the supported housing option. Marsha felt this would be the best option but Leon had been reluctant to leave.

"I had to be tough on Leon," she explained, reaching the point where she had the difficult task of telling him that she would evict him if he did not go to the supported accommodation. She then said with obvious relief: "Leon says he's happy now." On balance, she felt this had been the right course of action. "When they get the treatment right, everything will be back to normal. This illness takes patience."

Leon's transition from his mother's home into his own room at the supported accommodation project had been driven, to a significant extent, by Marsha's needs, in particular the impact on her health of being a carer for him. To illustrate the demands of this role, Farooq recounted a story from the previous year when Leon had locked himself inside, and Marsha out of, the family's flat. She had eventually managed to regain entry, but only with the assistance of the out-of-hours emergency duty team of social workers.

Leon's initial account of this incident, Farooq said, was that he had not heard Marsha buzzing or ringing. But when pressed about all the doors and windows being secured, Leon had begun, slowly, to talk about his mental distress and tendency to retreat into himself when facing pressures. This, Farooq felt, had opened up a space for dialogue between them that had been important in the development of his working relationship with Leon.

Nonetheless, Leon remained reluctant to move out. His mother was keen for this process to happen quickly and even threatened to take legal action to evict her son. Farooq tried to carefully balance these competing perspectives by beginning the work to facilitate the move, but also ensuring a carefully measured pace that acknowledged Leon's ambivalence and took seriously his concerns about managing the process and living independently. Leon refused, on a couple of occasions, to move on the date planned. Farooq finally managed to persuade him to agree during a long telephone call. Farooq felt that the avoidance of force and legal measures, while working with Leon's concerns and anxieties about the move, had been crucial factors in the final decision. The day after Leon's move, Farooq's demeanour had suggested a sense of satisfaction.

From this point onwards, Farooq described a reduction in the frequency of his meetings with Leon. He was visiting Leon "once every month or sometimes once every six weeks, it's kind of doing [a] CPA [Care Programme Approach] review [or] other stuff. But there isn't that much therapeutic relationship." He felt this was not "ideal" but a combination of higher levels of support for Leon at the residential setting and Farooq's other workload pressures determined this situation. These demands were predominantly bureaucratic, driven by targets, for instance "much more work around personal budgets".

One ongoing aspect of Farooq's role had been supporting Leon with his application to register for a college access course in digital design as a gateway to degree studies. Leon's application was initially turned down by the social care funding panel. But it was later granted when the application for funding was resubmitted, on the advice of the assistant director of social care, but this time using a personalisation approach via the personal budgets system. Farooq expressed frustration with the inconsistency evidenced by this scenario, and how outcomes now seemed driven by social care targets rather than service user need.

The significance of orderings of time is visible in these events. Farooq described the therapeutic temporality of building trust and exploring and supporting Leon around his concerns, while working slowly and carefully towards the move. For Farooq, this temporal ordering also enabled a consensual and negotiated approach between Leon, Marsha and other family members. This underlines the highly indeterminate nature of mental health work, involving negotiating and balancing between the needs of a variety of actors while also mobilising elements of practical, bureaucratic and emotional forms of labour. However, having prioritised support to Leon and intensified his time commitment in order to facilitate this transition, Farooq then had to withdraw and readjust to an informational temporality due to other demands on his caseload.

Ray

Just along the street from Leon's housing project was the mental health registered care home where Ray was a resident. Beside the imposing wood-panelled front door crowned by a fanlight arch window was a large intercom, although no signage outside to indicate the nature of this project. Having been buzzed into the building, I passed a cramped office located just to the right inside the door. On the day of my visit one project worker was sitting at the large desk, with another in a chair beside them.

The project housed 17 men with mental health needs, each with their own bedroom, and there were shared communal areas including a dining room and lounges. Several service users linked to Southville CMHT lived there, with the project catering for people with higher and longer-term levels of need, to which mental health workers sometimes attached the label "chronic". There were a couple of smaller meeting rooms opposite the office so that project staff and the many professionals visiting could meet with residents with a degree of privacy. A project worker led me into one of these spaces. It contained three soft chairs separated by a coffee table from two office chairs at a bench with two rather ancient-looking computers.

Ray was waiting for me there and greeted me with a handshake as the worker introduced us. I noticed Ray's hand trembling as he returned it to his side. Ray was a short and slim White British man with gaunt features and cropped grey hair, who looked at least a decade older than his 50 years. He smiled and greeted me chirpily in a strong cockney accent. On an earlier meeting with Ray and his care coordinator Leslie, the latter had commented on Ray's outgoing and humorous demeanour, describing him as a real "cheeky chappy". Ray had also shared at that meeting, however, that he typically drank three to four litres of cider a day. And sometimes, when "steaming drunk", he could become aggressive towards other residents and staff.

Ray said his mental health difficulties emerged early. "I was always worrying, even at the age of 12, giving myself stomach ulcers." A particular concern was literacy. "I used to pretend I could read and write," he explained. "I was lying through my teeth about it." As he progressed to his teenage years he described feeling depressed. "I didn't like myself. I was worrying about this and that, running away from it through drink."

At age 17 he was diagnosed with anorexia and bulimia. He attributed his issues with food to a desire to avoid gaining weight from the large quantities of alcohol he was drinking. He also described compulsive washing rituals: "It took me four hours to have a bath". From that point until he reached his 20s, Ray worked on the railways, but drinking was his priority. "I was wild in my 20s, denying it all, frustrated, why does it happen to me?"

In his 30s, he described things getting "really weird, desperate" and he started to hear voices. "I was like a radio DJ, talking away to the voices," he joked. "Initially they were cheerful voices but then they became aggressive." Ray described increasing his drinking "to fade away the voices. It worked a wee bit but it didn't do me any favours." As time went on, the voices started "shouting at me, do this, do that". As a result, one day, he started a fire in his house. A prison sentence followed. In the first year of his sentence, Ray's mother died. This was a significant low point for him. He described agonising over whether to attend the funeral, eventually deciding against it. "I didn't want to upset the family by going in handcuffs."

Ray was eventually transferred to a secure mental health forensic unit where he spent the next few years. In this unit he described how his psychiatrist "started me on the depots and I got well". But the trials with different medications had led him to feel at times like a "guinea pig". The side effects bothered him. "The jaw movements were embarrassing." As well as medication, he felt the psychiatrists he encountered were preoccupied with his drinking rather than the distress that precipitated it. "They should focus on the mental health, not so much on the alcohol."

Ray also had "a change of psychiatrist every six months, which was a pity because it takes a while to get to know your psychiatrist. I don't think that's right. You have to start from square one again, kind of repeating yourself." As a result, he did not know who the doctors were. That was frustrating, because "psychiatrists have got [an] understanding [of mental health], but they need to get to know the person properly."

Ray was eventually released from the forensic unit into the care of the CMHT. As well as changing his medication to reduce the side effects, he welcomed the more consistent relationships he had been able to access with CMHT practitioners, most recently his care coordinator Leslie. Ray said the practitioners "are doing more work now like psychiatrists used to. Leslie knows me better than the psychiatrist knows me." Ray was supportive of these changing professional roles: "I think it's a good idea to be honest." He described Leslie as "friendly [and] easy to talk to. And you have to get to know someone to feel more relaxed."

Leslie used narrative therapy to develop his working relationship with Ray. In one session, Leslie worked with Ray to construct a 'tree of life' diagram that mapped his hopes, strengths, aspirations and family connections. As a result, Ray later took steps to reconnect with his brother after a long estrangement since his spell in prison. Ray joked he would "sometimes run away" when he saw Leslie coming, then added in a more serious tone that the 'tree of life' had got him thinking. He reflected that, if he had been offered that kind of therapy in his 20s, he would probably have told Leslie to "fuck off". But now "I'm quite willing to talk. It gets me thinking, it feels good."

Leslie told me there were times Ray became more challenging. During one visit to the project, Ray had been physically threatening. Leslie was worried about violence and had had to talk Ray "very carefully out of the office". But Ray had telephoned him the next day, really apologetic and remorseful about the incident, saying that he had been "steaming" drunk. And, Leslie said, Ray mostly managed his alcohol use carefully.

Leslie went on to explain that, in view of Ray's decision to continue to use alcohol, he had decided not to focus on this issue in the work. "That's freed me up to look at his strengths," Leslie said. "He can be extremely self-critical and harsh on himself." Leslie thought narrative tools such as the 'tree of life' were a good way to facilitate this strengths focus. But it was harder and harder for him to do that kind of therapeutic work, because increasing caseloads meant the service was "bursting at the seams".

Ben

Ben's home was a cramped one-bedroom flat in a three-storey Victorian house on a busy thoroughfare with brickwork stained by decades of thick exhaust fumes from the seemingly endless flow of traffic. It was hard to make myself heard on the intercom because of the din from the engines and horns of slow-moving cars, delivery vans and lorries that inched their way forward behind me. When my shouts finally became audible during a rare gap between vehicles, I was buzzed in, and walked up a narrow flight of stairs.

Ben greeted me at his front door. He was tall and slim and looked younger than his 42 years, dressed in jeans, a t-shirt and a hooded top. Ben invited me into his small kitchen–dining area. I edged myself past dusty guitar amps, a portable audio mixing desk and piles of cardboard boxes of medical supplies. I lowered myself into a dining chair beside the round table in the middle of the room. The cacophony of traffic noise from below was somewhat muffled by the double-glazed door and window beside us that led onto Ben's narrow balcony. Ben explained that the housing association had recently replaced the windows and fittings in the flat and, although he found the weeks of disruption while the work was carried out draining, he was generally satisfied with the results. "They got the carpet colour wrong though!" he complained, but with comedic exaggeration.

As he joined me at the table, Ben pointed to the cold sores around his mouth and apologised for his appearance. "Vanity isn't good, but it's all I've got left," he said. Ben had suffered with significant pain and digestive problems for many years and had eventually been diagnosed with a severe form of Crohn's disease. As a result, he required regular appointments with a hospital consultant and attended numerous check-ups. These had become even more frequent recently as Ben had signed up to join a medical trial for a new treatment for this condition.

Ben had previously worked as a musician, just about earning a living. But since his physical health symptoms had intensified and the treatment commitments became more time-intensive he had given that up. He was also a painter and occasionally sold a piece of his artwork but did not earn enough from that to get by. Ben had been in contact with mental health services long before these physical health problems had become debilitating.

He said a diagnosis of bipolar disorder was "on my notes somewhere". But he was currently seeing the team "for major depressive disorder and anxiety".

Ben considered it essential not to conceptualise his physical and mental health experiences as somehow separate and unrelated. In particular, he felt the link between his experiences of pain and anxiety should be viewed in a holistic and integrative way. "They're interchangeable, that's the problem, and my case really displays it, how difficult it is to identify, is this an anxiety or is this a physical symptom? At the height of both, they become the same experience. But health systems struggle with conceptions of intertwined mental and physical health." Ben was interested in ideas from non-Western medicine, as he felt these more strongly recognised the "body–mind connection".

A major concern for Ben was that his current treatments for physical and mental health issues "contradicted" each other at times. Ben described an experience that, for him, illustrated this failure to recognise and implement a holistic approach. He had visited his general practitioner (GP) to discuss the pain he was experiencing because of Crohn's disease. Ben found it difficult to describe the pain to her, and felt the GP responded rather insensitively to his disclosure. She seemed unsympathetic to his experiences and the other anxieties about his health he tried to tell her about. She suggested that the pain associated with his condition might be "in the mind" and recommended cognitive behavioural therapy (CBT). He felt she did not believe him.

Other similar experiences reinforced Ben's sense that "as a patient I don't have much of a voice". For this reason, he considered it necessary for patients to assert, and practitioners to facilitate, a more active role in healthcare processes.

'You can't be passive. You have got to say to the doctor: "No, look, this symptom is happening like this." Otherwise what else does the doctor have apart from their discipline? That's all they can put on to it. You've got to be active enough for that to be the thing they listen to. And it's hard, it's hard as a physical patient. My physical problems have got scans, they've got blood tests, all this data to support it and its hard enough there to get understood as a patient, let alone with something as subjective and hard to quantify as a mental health problem.'

Some of his former psychiatrists had left Ben feeling that his experiences were not listened to or understood. He mentioned Dr Graham: "a suited, old-school biomedical" type, the kind of doctor who said, "you must have a chemical imbalance". Others, too, had been "stern" or made him feel "like a naughty schoolboy".

In contrast to these 'old-school' psychiatrists, Ben described Dr Bryant (James), his current consultant, as "very warm, very different. He makes the

patient feel at ease, is inclusive. He helps me to articulate [my experiences]."
Ben really valued James's support with this 'articulation' process and described several aspects of it. One was the way James helped him to describe and explore his experiences of pain and anxiety. Unlike the GP, James validated Ben's experiences.[5] The second dimension was that James "helped me to see the pattern of how, when I feel intimidated by someone, I struggle to articulate what I mean. He made the connection between that and my mother, when she becomes tyrant mother, and me not being able to flourish in those situations." Ben found it valuable to reflect on these intrapsychic identifications between his mother and the GP, who was also an older woman. Again, Ben felt this therapeutic exploration enabled better understanding of the intrapsychic barriers preventing articulation of his experiences.

A third significant aspect was that James had a more holistic approach to prescribing. Previous psychiatrists had prescribed Ben a variety of biomedical treatments, but James had been sensitive to the impact on his digestive tract. So now Ben was no longer on any psychotropic medications. As well as reducing potential digestive problems, Ben welcomed this because, as an artist and musician, he "didn't want to be dampened down". Consequently, Ben had reconsidered some of his previous misgivings about psychiatric support. "There's an area from which psychiatry is useful, about how people are coping with their physical problems and the wider implications and the reflection in their mental health."

Ben now thought the interface between physical and mental health was one area where psychiatry could be useful, provided the lived experiences and expertise of the patient were central in shaping and defining the understanding of and response to health issues. For this reason, Ben was somewhat dismissive of an older friend of his, Timothy, who was also a service user, and "extremely anti-psychiatry". While Ben disagreed with him, he could understand his friend's concerns because he had "gone through the dark days of psychiatry". Ben was referring to the electroconvulsive therapy (ECT) treatments Timothy had forcibly undergone during the 1960s. But he rejected his friend's view that all psychiatrists were the same. "That's not my experience of doctors," Ben said. He believed that, at least in principle, a better more holistic approach to psychiatry was possible. Ben then engaged in a thought experiment about what an alternative psychiatry might look like. "Mental health is a spectrum, and there are issues on both sides of the medicine trolley." So, his ideal psychiatrist would have personally experienced a mental health condition, and would be kept in check by the medical discipline, but have an empathy due to lived experience. Such a practitioner could "act as a translator between doctors and patients".

Still, there was at least one point of difference between Ben and James. Ben said that Dr Bryant had expressed reservations about his integrative mind–body philosophy of health, because of its potential to imply that the service user should accept causal culpability for their condition. "Are you blaming yourself for the illness?" James had asked Ben. In contrast, James defended the legitimacy of a 'sick role' position for his patients[6] at points of serious mental health crisis.

While Ben saw Dr Bryant at his outpatient clinic for an hour every three months, his care coordinator, social worker Constance, met with him on a monthly basis. Ben valued highly what he called her "ambient support". This was vital, because he needed "someone to talk to. Friends have a limit, and the pressure is not on them because of Constance." He thought the particular value of the care coordinator was a function of their unique positioning. "I can voice my concerns because she is not a doctor, and not a friend. Constance sees me in situ, in my native environment. It's more intimate." He was "a bit removed with Dr Bryant, more guarded. You have to be careful what you say to a doctor. I might say I feel suicidal to Constance but not to Dr Bryant or my friends."

He feared the emotional impact of such disclosures on friends. But with doctors it was partly the formality, but even more because "with one stroke of a pen he could make my life good or bad". Dr Bryant had the statutory power to make recommendations to detain him in hospital under Mental Health Act (MHA) legislation. Although Ben had never been detained under the Act, he described how these legal powers formed a tacit backdrop to their relationship. "I don't feel sectionable now, but that's not to say I'm not unaware of that dynamic."

However, Ben felt he was now receiving treatment on a different basis and the main issue was the impact of Crohn's disease on his mental health. He explained that this meant issues of power were less foregrounded, which was much better. Ben then reflected beyond his own situation to the wider implications of these power dynamics. "It's a big problem with those powers, it leads to a game of cat and mouse between psychiatrists and patients." Nonetheless, Ben felt there were some situations where potential harm would justify detention. He felt Timothy tended to minimise such dangers. Once, he challenged his friend: "You weren't sectioned because you were wearing the wrong trousers!"

The Crohn's disease diagnosis also impacted on the way causality was conceived in relation to his mental health. "Doctors can't just say chemical imbalance now. They have to acknowledge physical health. Even if we cure the chemical imbalance, I will still have things in my life that cause anxiety and depression ... I'm both lucky and unlucky that I have a physical marker that means that they can't just throw pills at me."

Constance broadly agreed with Ben's perspective. Her starting point was that "not being listened to had an impact on him feeling depressed". Instead of reinforcing this sense of invalidation, she argued for more relational and democratic practice. "You've got to have an understanding of the person, or you're just going to be another, you know, somebody who's just saying, no, well, you know, dictating how somebody's life should go."

This meant being there to listen to him, and for him to "use me as a sounding board". This was rooted in a strengths perspectives. In particular, she lauded Ben's strong orientation towards autonomy and self-management, in spite of his physical health. "He was determined, you know, 'I can do this, I can manage that'. It was a pleasure to have somebody who didn't, as much as there was a disability, didn't let that, there was something about him that still pushed on and you know, got on with it." Although this evokes a responsibilising self-care discourse, overall Constance was oriented to creating the conditions for "mutual respect". But she also described certain limits to this position, or what might be called a 'conditional trust' position (Brown and Calnan, 2012):

'So, Dr Bryant would kind of give him something to help him sleep. There was a time in Ben's life when he was an addict. So he would talk to me and when he said, "Oh, I need to see Dr Bryant", it wasn't often, but that would always happen and I used to think: "Hmm, is this to do with you not being able to sleep?" I don't know if that's bad, but it did cross my mind a few times, I didn't know if he was spinning me. It was there but, you know, he was fine. It was nothing that I thought there's a risk, but it was something that, had he kept persisting in that direction, then I would have had to go down and start looking at what's going on here.'

This reflects the tensions surrounding the trust–control dialectic in professional practice. But Constance was keen to maintain, as far as possible, a stance rooted in an 'atmosphere of trust' in anticipation of the destabilising and demoralising potentials of a more risk-oriented approach.

At the same time as Ben felt the support from the team was increasingly sensitive to his needs, his distress intensified due to reduced levels of support because of austerity-related retrenchment. He received a letter to say that Constance would no longer be working with him. "It was due to the cuts," he said. "Budgets have been slashed. It's a shame." He worried that Dr Bryant's support would be cut or reduced next. Ben would have liked at least a telephone call from Constance. But he acknowledged the pressure on workers. "They are being pushed to the limit, being asked to do ten times as much for half as little."

Harriet

Harriet was a small-framed woman in her late 50s. When I first met her I was struck by her purposeful stride, shoulders pushed back as she entered the room. Harriet wore a smart green quilted jacket and large round glasses, her fine straggly hair tied back to reveal a round face with a slightly ruddy complexion. She spoke quickly, introducing herself with impeccable manners and a confidence that indicated familiarity with the rituals of polite conversation.

Harriet had used mental health services for almost 30 years. Her first contact was when she experienced a "florid attack" at the age of 27. She spent three months in a psychiatric hospital. This was a highly traumatic event for both Harriet and her parents. She was close to them, and still living at home. After her discharge she was referred on to community mental health services, and returned to her "steady" job, an administrative role in a high-street bank.

After "a good long gap", another "attack" led to a second hospital admission. After that, Harriet had another six admissions to hospital. The psychiatric diagnosis she was given in these earlier stages was schizophrenia, but over the years this changed to schizoaffective disorder, "and I think it's now bipolar". As the label changed, the treatment plan evolved too. Harriet had been prescribed depot injections of Modecate for many years, but on her request this was eventually changed to tablets, currently the antipsychotic olanzapine.

Our discussion soon turned to the causes of mental distress. Harriet paused momentarily to reflect on the nature of relationships with her family and firmly discounted that as a factor. While the loss of a friend to suicide at university had been difficult, she did not think that was the cause either. She settled on the idea that causal factors are multiple and hard to discern. "That's one of the most difficult things, because people long to say: 'Oh, it's because of such and such.' Unfortunately, you have to realise that in the end it might be a bit of a mystery and you might never find it." So Harriet felt there was little therapeutic utility in "digging for the cause in the past". Instead, focusing on factors in the present, in particular strengthening interpersonal support, were paramount. "Picking yourself up is about, take you where it's at, and try to form a new relationship of steadiness."

To illustrate the importance of what she called the "human stuff", Harriet talked about her distress during one of her hospital admissions. "I can remember being very angry with [staff] who were saying: 'Oh, can I give you a drug to calm you down.' Whereas [another nurse] put off what [their] other duty was. They'd sit on my bed and hold my hand, and the human stuff that many nurses are afraid to practise because of risk assessment."

Harriet explained in detail the most important aspects of relational support. In doing so she indicated the importance of mutual interaction between these elements. Her starting point was the importance of re-establishing "steadiness and stability". Harriet noted that in the initial stages of the crisis, "friends will find you more and more demanding. They want to meet you, but they can't cope."

As a result, Harriet was left:

'in a position of loneliness, and not a great many other places where there are friends who would support me through a crisis. So the practitioner is absolutely vital. And I think that in the first experience of the client of considerable and humbling vulnerability, and inability to cope, the practitioner must take their first steps to establishing a relationship, a trusting relationship.'

For Harriet, trust was a core requirement of interpersonal engagements because "one of the aspects of my childhood is just not trusting anybody outside the family". So this was integral to making it work with a practitioner. "If they go rushing in enthusiastically and say, 'Now you're going to swim five times a week', the patient says, 'I'm not going back there again', and they never do. Then, the practitioner has lost them."

Harriet thought that consistency and continuity of support over time were "vital".

'If a patient sees a different person each time, it's like reinventing the wheel. A new practitioner has got to establish the ground level of trust from which to take the thing forward, and the patient arguably in the end says, "Oh, for god's sake, I've said this so many times" ... But if a patient does experience [trust with a practitioner], and they want it enough, they will go on coming back for it, because it's a marvellous thing to have been on the receiving end of.'

The dominant contemporary policy discourse asserts that there is a risk of dependency arising from such longer-term relationships with community workers (Brown and Baker, 2012). However, Harriet described the support she received as varying from more to less frequent according to her needs over time. As she explained:

'For a long time I only needed a three-monthly meeting. After the emergence of a crisis, and more regular help being needed, somebody like Evelyn would take over. I'd see them every two weeks. If I came out of hospital and I needed more input, then it would be available to me.'

Moreover, Harriet did not think there was a conflict between extended support and her self-defined goal of "finding self-reliance". Current arrangements were enabling her to achieve this aim. "My ability to be self-reliant has come from somewhere in the help that I've received. In my case, I am lucky that it's been one [Evelyn] for a very long time." Harriet's perspective presents a challenge to the neoliberal 'common sense' around minimising longer-term support to reduce dependency. In her countervailing orientation, greater independence was conceptualised as an emergent property of longer-term therapeutic support.

But Harriet knew the kind of arrangements from which she had benefitted were under threat. The increasing emphasis on short-term, time-limited support meant that "continuity of any sort is becoming quite a luxury. Nevertheless, it is incredibly important." The new short-term approaches were a "firefighting situation". Services were reduced to "have a diagnosis, a dealing and the shortest of possible help".[7] That was "so much less good than what we have here".

What Harriet valued in the relational work took place not only in individual casework but also in "community building" spaces. Harriet had first met Evelyn through their mutual involvement in the 'My Story' narrative workshops. Harriet spoke very warmly about narrative approaches. She said that they place "the person as the expert in their own life". Harriet explained that My Story events were open to all involved in the Trust – "for people who are ill, their carers and nurses, and the introductions do not make clear which you are". That challenged hierarchical role demarcations: "If you are a patient, and you are a parent, and you can't talk to your own, or you are a patient and you are a practitioner, and it's difficult to cross [those boundaries], the My Story group somehow is a brilliant design."

Harriet took an increasing interest in narrative therapy and began reading more widely on it. Using the terminology of this perspective, Harriet became more critical of certain aspects of standard service provision. She said of the therapeutic pessimism of the medical model that "a diagnosis and a dismal outlook is a thin description".[8]

Instead, narrative practice enabled her to construct "a thick description" in her own life. That was "such a breath of fresh air. One of the desperate things about depression is the vicious circle, and one of the things about narrative therapy is the virtuous circle of bringing a story out of it and taking the thing onto a new level." With the encouragement of Evelyn and others, she then began to take a more active role in My Story. It became "an important part of every aspect of my life. And occasionally I co-present it and take a part" in running the sessions.

When Evelyn later became Harriet's care coordinator, their joint interest in narrative therapy shaped the nature of their work together. For Harriet, the theoretical ideas underpinning this perspective, what she called the "structured stuff", were important. But "the human stuff is completely vital. And the structured stuff, it must use the human stuff." Harriet did not think relational support was just about practitioners. Mutual support among service users mattered a great deal. "The experience that people have among themselves is something that they give each other forever, based on, 'yes, I've been there'. The friendships you make can be very deep." But relational support was an essential and urgent task far beyond that. "Community building needs to be done absolutely everywhere in the world at the moment. It's priority number one."

One of the most difficult aspects of Harriet's mental health crisis had been losing her job in a bank after 22 years' service. This was not her choice. "And it took a long time for the universe to find another centre. If you aren't successful in personal emotional relationships, then work is really crucial in defining you to yourself." Harriet lost friends, and "really dreaded life without the format that I was used to ... One big thing to counteract the loneliness is identifying oneself in a positive way. Narrative therapy has been important for this."

Harriet found the increasing emphasis on back-to-work and recovery agendas in recent mental health policy problematic. In particular, she pointed to the challenge of discrimination in the labour market. "One of the discouraging aspects when applying for a job, is the fact that a new employer would not have any notion that the person was reliable from the fact that they have a mental history as long as mine. I am, as it happens, pretty reliable." This also implicitly devalues other social roles such as volunteering work. Harriet said she no longer finds the stigma of not being employed debilitating. Now she can "say proudly I've got four voluntary roles". One of these is campaigning and advocacy work on mental health with a large third sector organisation. "After the second admission I decided to get really involved, make it an important part of my life."

Another multilayered tension for Harriet was her use of medication. "When there's a state of crisis, it is about medication and prevention of relapse. And medication is second to none really." During difficult moments she was willing to accept prompts from people she trusted.

> 'When Evelyn has had to tell me, "Harriet, you've got to start taking your pills again", she knows how to do it. She'll lead me in gently. But that is because we have a relationship now where she can do that. But it never fails to disappoint me that what people really come back to forever is medication. I have organised my life really so that I have as little of them as possible, really only PRN [pro re nata, that is, only as needed] now. I do wish that I had not said yes for 30 years to taking them, because I have lost so many brain cells. I have experience of what is early dementia. I'm saying a sentence and I can't find the word, and that makes me so angry.'

Harriet thought her psychiatrists would not approve of this self-imposed strategy to limit medication use. For them, antipsychotic medication was regarded as a necessary ongoing treatment to prevent 'relapse'. As she explained:

> 'I think a dilemma might always be the temptation to say: "If I say I'm taking this they'll go away" ... I'm afraid that probably continues to be a deception. If anybody, apart from the practitioner in question, asked me, I'll say: "Would you mind leaving that between me and my practitioner?" And if my practitioner asks me, I should probably say: "Well, [coughs] I kind of am." And in the end I'll say: "Look, you have to leave it to me to be the judge." There are many practitioners to whom I could not say it.'

Harriet also described similar dilemmas about her "hallucinatory experiences ... It's about self-preservative boundaries. If this nurse, to whom I tell this, is about to lock me up, common sense says, the fragment of common sense still remains, just don't tell them this bit". This highlights how issues of trust and the service user's decision making around their treatment are embedded within wider relations of power.

Harriet concluded by describing the precariousness of services in the face of 20 per cent cuts that the Trust had recently announced. These funding constraints reflected the wider policy agenda of austerity.

> 'If it was simply an accountant coming in and saying, "It costs too much", if an accountant says, "Can you save 20 per cent", actually they may destroy the whole thing. They say we're going to have less, and we're going to do more with it. ... Actually in the end everybody does crack, because in the end they're doing six jobs where they were doing one, and half the ship has gone, and the people you want have gone, and the people who are left can't cope. In mental health it really wouldn't work because you've got to have reliability. Patients are in need of care, some peace and reliable stuff.'

Harriet was extremely complimentary about the support she received from Evelyn. She expressed gratitude for Evelyn's assistance in the process of coming off Modecate, an older antipsychotic medication taken by injection, which had been her primary treatment for many years.

Evelyn talked about that too:

> 'We kind of did that together and I suppose we reduced Modecate very slowly, over about a year I was really pleased about the way that that all worked out. Then she transferred to some oral medication. Harriet's really taught me to sort of go with your instincts, because

I was just like, I thought, "Well, I'm not sure this is doing any good, this medication", you know, and to go with what the client says that they want.'

This user-centred approach had contributed to the development of a good rapport between them, and this was reinforced by Evelyn's advocacy on Harriet's behalf, particularly around medication. As Evelyn noted, Harriet's 'as and when needed' way of using her current oral medication was something that her psychiatrists did not "necessarily approve of". But Evelyn supported Harriet in defending this strategy with doctors. "We agreed that we would do it the way that she wanted to."

This emphasis on relational and reciprocal forms of practice was also visible in the contrast Evelyn drew between tick-box 'informational' approaches and 'real' CMHT work. She argued that both she and Harriet were strongly oriented to the latter. She said that Harriet:

'Would be quite happy to have a template tick-box care plan that we did. And then that's that and then we get down to the real business, which is about our relationship and about what [she] wants and you know, what I can help with, and what would be helpful and how we intend to work together.'

Evelyn compared herself to McNulty in the television drama *The Wire*, whose philosophy involved "fudging things a little bit, just to get the organisation off our back". It was a necessary tactic to preserve spaces for work outside of the agenda defined by the organisational target culture. But Evelyn knew that her scope to carve out such discretionary spaces was, to some degree, a function of her seniority. "I've always had a certain amount of kind of clinical freedom as a team manager. People don't tend to question what I do." She laughed.

This collaborative ethos was also apparent in Evelyn's encouragement to Harriet to increase her involvement with the My Story workshops and become an expert-by-experience consultant and trainer. Both Harriet and Evelyn identified with the democratic orientation of narrative approaches, which challenge established constructions of professional boundaries rooted in the medical model. This highlights the value placed on the mutuality, friendly relationships and humanity of workers, while the relational and reciprocal nature of such professional relationships offers psychological benefits to the worker as well as the service user (O'Leary et al, 2013). This may account for the sense of loss described by CMHT workers as these new informational service arrangements began to dominate.

Evelyn was also critical of another element of the recent reform agenda in CMHTs: the increasing 'back-to-work' focus:

'When people meet Harriet, then they think, "Well, she could be doing something useful." Well, I believe she *is* doing something incredibly useful. One, she's protecting her mental health and two, she's doing all the voluntary work that she does. But it's kind of like getting people to step back from this idea that it's just about paid employment, and stopping [psychiatrists] putting too much pressure on her to recover, in terms of going and getting work.'

For Evelyn, this focus was linked with wider notions of welfare dependency associated with service use: "This whole concept of dependency, it kind of needs deconstructing because it's seen as a very bad thing and you know, but we're all dependent on each other, aren't we?"

Trust and relational practice at Southville CMHT

These case studies highlight the value placed by the service users on empathy, respect and being listened to in their relationships with practitioners (Beresford et al, 2008). Val, Ben and Harriet also emphasised qualities of professional competence and an ethical approach to practice. But the service users could see emerging threats to such values. Harriet and Ben noted the impact of the austerity agenda and its effects on levels of support from practitioners. Val, Jorge and Ray expressed concern about the harmful effects of neoliberal reforms such as outsourcing and short-term service provision, which reduced the consistency and continuity of care. Jorge, Ray, Ben and Harriet also disagreed with the over-emphasis on medication. Ben drew attention to the way this undermined trust (Vassilev and Pilgrim, 2007; Szmukler and Rose, 2013).

These service users also disagreed on some things. Val saw some legitimacy in medical paternalism. But Ben advocated the autonomy and expertise of the service user as a core philosophy that should underpin provision regardless of individual circumstances. Harriet too foregrounded expertise from lived experience. However, she made the case for a more integrative position that balances the need for expertise by experience and maintaining a role for and placing value on expertise by profession. This highlights the importance of developing alliances in user–professional relationships, an approach that chimed with that of all the care coordinators included here (Nutt and Keville, 2016). This has affinities with Lethbridge's (2019) notion of 'democratic professionalism', where structures of public service provision are rooted in mutual trust, based on egalitarian, empathic forms of service user–professional engagement, and oriented to control by service users. That is certainly how Evelyn and Leslie tried to work.

The service users introduced in this chapter generally valued and advocated relational approaches as an organising principle for provision. However, the practitioners talked about the negative impact of the informational turn on connections with service users. Nonetheless, they sought to protect and extend relational spaces in spite of the informational and temporal pressures associated with neoliberal reconfigurations.

4

Risk and responsibilisation

The last chapter introduced a number of service users and practitioners. The examples described relational casework during what practitioners called a 'stable phase' and challenges to this associated with new informational ways of working. This and the next chapter build on and extend this exploration of the dialectic of possibility and constraint in CMHT work through a focus on interactions with service users considered to be 'in crisis'. This chapter is about Emmanuel, or Manu as he is generally known to family members and practitioners, and his experiences at Southville CMHT and within inpatient services. It illustrates how a defensive institutional culture around risk management generates tendencies towards what is called 'custodial paternalism'. It also examines how this marginalises considerations on the effects of racialised inequalities.

Upton Ward at the Middletown Centre Mental Health Unit

Many of the events in this chapter took place on 'Upton' Ward, part of the 'Middletown Centre' Mental Health Unit at 'Westside Park' Hospital[1]. The hospital is an NHS facility providing adult and older persons' mental health in-patient services. It is located on a site encompassing several imposing red-brick buildings, constructed as a workhouse infirmary in the late Victorian era. Upton Ward has 16 beds, eight for men and the same number for women in a separate area.

Every week there is a ward round. This is a multidisciplinary meeting on Monday mornings where Upton Ward staff meet with each individual patient, community team members and, where possible, informal carers such as family members, to explore the patient's progress and review and develop care plans. This is generally led by the consultant psychiatrist. During the fieldwork, this meeting took place in a room halfway between the nurses' station and the lounge. Eight or nine chairs were placed in a large circle for the meeting, with any spares stacked at the side of the room. The spring on the room's heavy door meant that it slammed every time someone entered or left and, in combination with resin flooring and high Victorian ceilings, the sound echoed piercingly around the space. The faint sound of a Bollywood playback singer drifted in from one of the bedrooms. Consultant psychiatrist Dr James Bryant insisted the chair next to him be left solely for patients to use, complaining that he struggled to hear what was said otherwise.

Manu

Manu is a 23-year-old Black British man. His parents settled in the UK from Nigeria before he was born. Manu has been subject to the intensive involvement of psychiatric services since his teenage years, when he was first admitted to a mental health unit. He has spent much of the intervening period in contact with services, and most of the last three years as an inpatient on various psychiatric wards in the Trust. Manu hears voices that are critical of him and he finds this experience deeply distressing. He has been given the diagnostic label of schizophrenia. When I first met Manu he had just begun the process of transferring from Upton Ward to the 'Britchcombe Road' Hostel, a local community-based residential project.

Treatment and intervention

This section examines the evolving care plan and then the contrasting understandings of Manu's mental health and accommodation needs as articulated by Manu himself and the various professionals and teams working with him. The most prominent of these are James, his consultant psychiatrist, and Abbie, his community mental health nurse and care coordinator. As we will see, there were significant differences in their understandings of how to work with Manu.

Ward round 1

James typically had about half a dozen patients to see during his ward round. This week Manu was the third. Some consultants were known to try to work through patients as quickly as possible, but James was not one of these. He sometimes took three quarters of an hour or more for each patient. Most Community Mental Health Team (CMHT) members valued his willingness to spend this time talking with patients. But some reported that others (although not themselves) were less keen. This may be a consequence of the amount of time out from their busy schedules involved in making the half an hour journey from the CMHT to the Middletown Centre and then, often, waiting for the turn of the service user they care coordinated.

Manu was in the process of transferring from Upton Ward to Britchcombe Road Hostel, as already noted, but had not yet been formally discharged. He still returned to the ward several nights a week, with a plan for a gradual reduction. However, Manu had been discharged from Section 3 of the Mental

Health Act 2007 (MHA) under which he had been detained on Upton Ward and placed on a community treatment order (CTO). On this Monday ward round, staff were hopeful that the transition to the hostel could soon be completed. When Abbie arrived and checked in with the nurses in the office, she discovered Britchcombe Road staff had telephoned to say Manu was refusing to come to the meeting. Meanwhile, inside the ward round meeting, discussion with the previous patient was drawing to a close, and word of the 'no show' had just filtered through to the consultant James from a ward nurse. Exasperated, James said: "He's on a CTO, he can't refuse to come. That's not a good start." Many others had now arrived. "There's loads of us", Abbie observed as they entered the meeting room. "But no Manu", James replied with a hint of irritation.

Following Abbie in to the meeting was Manu's mother, then Martina, a support worker from Britchcombe, and Liz, an occupational therapist based at the Middletown Centre. Also present were a ward nurse, a student nurse, a junior doctor who typed a record for the RiO database on a laptop, and me. James began by asking why Manu had not come.

Martina explained that Manu was aware that Britchcombe staff had wanted to discuss concerns about his behaviour. She thought maybe he was avoiding the meeting for this reason. "Or maybe not even aware of this, maybe he was trying to sabotage this placement. Maybe he feels more safety here. Maybe it was too big a step for him. A bit too fast."

Martina explained the hostel's concerns. Manu was not coming to the project on some days even though this was what he was telling ward staff. At other times, there were complaints from hostel residents that he was stealing their food, and this continued even after he was supported to do his own shopping. Manu then claimed others were taking his food.

Martina thought maybe "at the beginning we were expecting too much from him, because as I said, most of our clients are older than Manu, most of them are on a section. So they are aware that if something goes wrong, they are going back to hospital or prison."

Martina continued by adding that he failed three or four times to go to a meeting with the activity coordinator about college courses, and "disappeared" when he was supposed to meet with a drug project. Project residents and staff felt "shock at the beginning that he's so unrespectful to the rules and the house rules and the contract which was signed," continuing that "he breached conditions and [the] licence agreement because he was smoking cannabis in his room, not even outside". Martina suggested slowing down the transition and using the CTO to reinforce "lots of conditions and things".

James explained the terms of the CTO, but then changed focus to examine the tension between Manu and residents at the project. James emphasised that Manu was very different from the kind of service user who was typically under a forensic section of the MHA:

'If they do anything very well, people on section 41 [of the MHA], they're very good at knowing what boundaries to stick to and this is a problem with Manu and has been for a long time, that he just pushes boundaries and he's quite immature in that respect. So, although he's in his 20s, he behaves like somebody who's 16 or 17 in that respect. I think that his development, his maturation, has been slowed down by the early onset of his mental illness and the long periods of institutionalisation, so he hasn't really taken on responsibility for himself. He's a bit like a teenager.'

While noting the impact of the social process of institutionalisation, James also speculated on a biological dimension. He explained that Manu had a "limited capacity for forward planning and forward thinking". James wondered whether this was:

'a symptom of schizophrenia, a cognitive change to do with reducing, you know, what we might call frontal lobe-type activity, frontal lobe-type thinking. So it may be that somehow, over time, that has to be compensated for. If Manu was in the forensic system and been seeing a psychologist for years, it would help him with that. At the moment, my impression is Manu's engagement with talking-type approaches is superficial. So he'll meet you and if he's in a good mood, he'll agree with everything you say and it feels quite shallow engagement. You don't really know how much has stuck, how much has been processed.'

In view of these multiple social and biological factors, James argued that things would most likely be difficult for Britchcombe Road Hostel for a while. He suggested ways of working with Manu in view of this type of need:

'There isn't a simple solution to it. He's got to develop and mature over time, but to have I think some boundaries beyond which you will not shift, but other boundaries which perhaps you're able to negotiate with him, so that he has to engage in negotiation, he learns about negotiation, but then also understands there are some absolutes which are non-negotiable. You have to say: "Well, you can't continue to live here if you continue to smoke cannabis in your room."'

James also advised the project to incorporate positive reinforcement, to be "energetically encouraging perhaps, not setting up too many pass–fail points, ones he'll fail, fail, fail, fail". Liz, the occupational therapist, then interjected to support this view, arguing for activities that would be motivating and enjoyable for Manu. James agreed and added, in response to

Martina's stipulation earlier in the meeting that Manu engage with a local substance misuse project, "I think appointments to see the drug services is important. I suppose also equally important are appointments to do nice things". However, Martina's position did not shift perceptibly in response to this. She was not optimistic about the outcome of the transition. "I can imagine that if it would be a few warnings from the management then he could be evicted."

James responded:

'But that's a reality as well and that's a reality none of us can necessarily take steps to avoid; it's in Manu's hands. He understands on some level that if he doesn't do it, well, that's a consequence. He'll be back at the beginning and I imagine back in hospital for a long time and that's a tragedy for him personally but, you know, we live and work in the world as it is and we can't wish that different.'

While evoking this argument around Manu taking responsibility for 'consequences', James and Liz also quickly returned to their efforts to try to encourage Martina to adopt a more hopeful stance. James continued:

'I mean, Manu, I suppose our experience is that Manu's adherence to boundaries has improved here, hasn't it? … It took a long time but towards the end, he has been an awful lot better … He's stuck to his leave conditions and I think it actually did help us when he had the goal of coming to you [Britchcombe Road] as a positive incentive and maybe that's what he needs again, you know, a meaningful daytime activity.'

Martina maintained her stance, then introduced the matter of Manu not taking his medication. The extent to which this constituted a key point of leverage in these negotiations was evident in James's response. He conceded that it "goes without saying, yeah, he'd have to be recalled pretty quickly if he stopped taking his medication". Martina reinforced these concerns: "If he's not taking meds and smoking cannabis, that's when he can be quite aggressive."

At this point, Abbie finally came in. She started by agreeing that Manu appeared to be "testing his limits" with Britchcombe Road. Then she supported Martina:

'When I met with Manu the other day, I was really struck, I felt really exhausted afterwards and he just seemed so angry. You know, there was no eye contact, we had to ask for that. I just felt this overwhelming sense of anger coming from him. It was very difficult.'

James sounded surprised, and curtly asked what Manu was angry with her about. It went "unsaid", but was apparent in the "non-verbals", she replied.

Martina returned to a similar theme shortly after: "The problem is with his lack of motivation or, he does not want to engage too much at our place. As I said, we have a lot of problems with this transition. Whatever we are trying to do this way or that way, it seems to not be working."

James seemed frustrated:

'I understand where you're coming from, but I suppose our experience is that over time, it does get easier, so give him time, you know. I would expect that this is the hardest point and it'll get easier from here, but obviously there are risks and he loses, you know, the tenancy, you know, he could get into trouble with another resident along the way. You know, these are risks and we have to be mindful of that and if he's not taking medication, we'll have to recall him to hospital.'

This plea by James emphasised the case for temporal flexibility and perseverance on the part of Britchcombe Road, and the need to give Manu time to settle and build relationships, as had been required before when he was a patient on the ward. James described medication, boundaries and encouragement as the three core dimensions enabling progress during his inpatient stay, implying that this was a realistic and feasible plan for Britchcombe Road to implement.

Abbie's perspective, part 1

And there the matter was left, for the time being. It had not been easy for Abbie to disagree with James in the ward round. The power differential between consultant psychiatrists and nurses remains significant, a legacy of the development of health service institutions as medically dominated hierarchies. This has both class and gendered dimensions. But Abbie felt it was important to express her view.

Defining service user needs

I interviewed Abbie a year later, as I was ending my fieldwork. One of the things we talked about was Manu's case. My understanding of her views comes from what she told me then. Her description of Manu's needs was framed by her perception of the risks he posed:

'We've had this tremendous violent history and he's still doing drugs like it's water ... We had a failed placement at Britchcombe Road and he was just completely psychotic, paranoid, unable to cope, had a big knife in his bedroom, told people it was because he was making baguettes, I mean, how awful is that? He threatened a pregnant worker, a *pregnant* worker, about doing her child in. He, ah, he stole a bicycle, which they lend, he borrowed a bicycle and went off and sold it. It was horrendous and the staff were like, within two weeks, scared out of their minds and they just insisted he went back on the ward.'

In her view this necessitated a different kind of plan, with an end to interminable discussions about hostels because, she explained, "he's going to die in a hostel, the man's going to be knifed or stabbed or something".

Abbie had been trained to use her feelings in developing insight in her work. She used this approach with Manu.

'I felt bored within six months, I just thought: "What's this, what are we doing, we're going round and round and round in a bloody great circle" … It's interesting, I think I work a bit differently, in that I listen to my feelings, right. And the thing was, I got desperation. There's all this desperation, try this hostel, try that hostel, you know. I contacted about 17 places and I just thought: "What is this, what is this?" I'm bored on the one hand and I'm stressed, you know, I'm feeling everyone else's panic about this guy. So, it was the combination and then I read the risk assessments and it was staring me in the face, he's forensic.'

This approach to mental health work, she explained, was rooted in her nursing training. This professional education instilled in her a sense that her 'self', her personality and her interpersonal skills represent the essential practice resources.

'My training was a one-year course. It was not particularly name, age and diagnosis, it was about developing your personality. So it is my personality, this is what I've got to offer the service user. This is me and that's it … There were eight people in the group. Most of the teaching was in a circle, so it was all like a group, all day long. It was about your skills – can you do it? And any problem you had would come out on that course, because it wasn't just sit and do an essay, it was like tasks, it was inner resources. And if I was a massive psychopath, it would have shown and if I had a psychosis, that would have come out, and if I'd have had a problem, it would have come out.'

This education served as a kind of laboratory for 'abnormal' mental states in the participants. This was, presumably, to ensure these were identified and treated, or filtered out of the profession. In his ethnography of psychiatric teamwork, Barrett (1996) notes the way in which nurses operate at much closer proximity to the more intense forms of mental distress than any other practitioner group. In such circumstances, the careful monitoring for and guarding against the signs of such distress within this professional group perhaps represent a type of splitting defence against such intimate interaction with the 'pathological'.

Abbie described two 'breakthroughs' in her work with Manu. The first was identifying the importance of 'personality' factors.[2] In practice, this meant a decision by her to investigate the possibility that Manu would meet the criteria for a diagnosis of personality disorder, an issue that had not been previously explored. Abbie explained that she had experienced a 'feeling' about it and so referred Manu to the personality unit at the local Mental Health In-Patient Centre for assessment. This process resulted in the identification of 'antisocial personality disorder' traits.

In achieving recognition of the role of Manu's personality traits, Abbie felt she had made a significant contribution to the process of 'moving on' the understanding and definition of his needs. Abbie defined herself as "a dynamic worker. When I saw nothing's changing, nothing's moving on, he's been like this for three years ... it's the sense of like agitation and I think by that I mean undynamic. Where's the dynamic, where's the changes, where's the structure?"

Abbie considered herself and her intervention a catalyst for change beyond an explanation for Manu's problems that saw them simply as rooted in psychosis and drug use, "into acknowledging he's got a serious personality disorder, drugs are like water, he's got a serious psychosis and he needs intense, intense care". Here, Abbie was at pains to emphasise the level and intensity of need. This not only implied the inappropriateness of the hostel referral but also provided justification for a different kind of intensive support and supervision plan. This was the other 'breakthrough', predicated on the attribution of antisocial personality traits but in combination with the risk factors already articulated by Abbie, which was to identify Manu as 'forensic'.

Abbie's use of this notion was based on the contradictory feelings she described in relation to the work with Manu. On the one hand, the process felt stuck and she had a sense of boredom. On the other, a highly charged emotional atmosphere was swirling around Manu, evoked by terms such as 'desperation', 'stress' and 'panic'. Recognising and buffeted by these countervailing dynamics of boredom and intensity, Abbie used her awareness of these, together with further consideration of risk and the written and oral narratives regarding Manu's behaviours, to re-evaluate the situation.

'It was reading the risk assessments over and over and over again, it was the feeling of repetitiveness, this is like really, because it just felt wishy-washy, you know. And then it was this desperation about accommodation, and what those feelings told me was that someone had missed it. For me, it was like, he's forensic, that's the point and he goes to a forensic unit and that's the problem with the accommodation, because no one will have him and this is the problem with the boredom, because you're treating it all wrong.'

Abbie identified what she saw as the most significant problem with the plan for Manu. He was being *treated* inappropriately and her problems in placing him were the evidence for this.

This account is particularly noteworthy because of the attention it directs towards Abbie's use of her feelings. This is no longer oriented, as it once might have been, towards the relationship with the service user and the use of self as a therapeutic tool in interpersonal interaction and a fulcrum around which the therapy revolves. Instead, while Abbie's feelings remained an interpretive apparatus for her, in this context they were used to gauge institutional rather than interpersonal dynamics. When she described her work it predominantly involved bureaucratic practices such as liaising with other services, completing accommodation application forms and, in particular, reading risk assessments. In so far as she engaged in direct interaction with Manu this took the form of attending formal meetings where he was also present, such as ward rounds and tribunal meetings. As such, her direct therapeutic engagement with him was limited by his status as an inpatient, and the bureaucratic and organisational demands placed on her. Her use of feelings, therefore, functioned as a barometer of institutional rather than interpersonal processes.

Moreover, it is notable that the 'desperation' and panic described came, in the main, not from Manu and his family or the immediate team working with him. A primary source of panic was the Accommodation Team, who subjected Abbie to what she described as "mountains of harassment". This pressure was rooted in a managerialist requirement to find a suitable accommodation placement for Manu to enable his discharge from the ward at the earliest possible opportunity after three years as a patient. Abbie's judgement concerning the definition of Manu's needs was thus shaped by her experience of this organisational context. Abbie had described numerous rejections from projects who were unwilling to accept Manu's referral, and in the context of increasing pressure on her to resolve this impasse, she considered this 'forensic' re-evaluation of his needs to be a breakthrough. For Abbie, the notion of 'forensic' was no longer merely an administrative label but was reconstituted as a form of diagnostic category.

Ward round 2

One week later, and this time Manu had made the journey to Westside Park Hospital for the ward round. He was accompanied by Aaron, the deputy manager from Britchcombe Road Hostel Many of the same professionals were present. So were Manu's mother and Mohinder, a senior psychiatric registrar (ST5) who worked with James. They were all drawn by a sense of gathering concern about the placement. Before Manu was invited to join, the practitioners and mother gathered in the meeting room. Asked for an update by James, Aaron's response followed a pattern similar to Martina's seven days before.

Aaron began with an incident over the weekend when there was suspicion that Manu was under the influence of cannabis:

'He'd been drinking and been stoned. He wasn't caught smoking but the behaviours were consistent with it ... Manu was in a very distressed state apparently and said that he was hearing voices telling him to kill a woman and a baby and then, on the following night, he was stating that he will kill a Black Ghanaian man from the staff who was working last week. Also, during the week, one of the sharp knives, there are two sharp knives per kitchen, which are checked daily, one of the sharp knives went missing and it was later found in his room. You know they are not allowed to take knives out of the kitchen and also there was some concern regarding his mental health, the command hallucinations, the threats, the knife going missing and also of course his previous history of threats.'

James paused for a moment, then said: "And tell us about the negatives." Aaron laughed anxiously.

James went on to ask about Manu's antipsychotic medication. He was told it had been declined on one occasion. James asked a junior doctor to check the drug chart and urged Britchcombe Road staff to be patient. He explained to Aaron that a pattern of 'pushing the boundaries' had been a feature of Manu's presentation at the hospital for some time. But, once Manu had eventually developed trust with people, things had "settled down an awful lot".

Aaron said there had been reports that Manu had not had enough money for food over the weekend in spite of a substantial benefits payment only days before. James floated the idea of appointeeship:

'If he's spending his money on drugs when actually he's not able to sustain himself, not eating and drinking and he's not taking care of himself, then I would say that we try and get some control over the money situation, which along the way could potentially benefit his drug habit.'

James paused again. Then he asked Jean-Paul, the ward nurse, if there were any beds. James had not discussed his decision with other staff, but this was a signal he had reluctantly accepted the need to bring Manu back onto the ward.

He went on to reflect on these developments, apparently thinking out loud rather than addressing anyone in particular. "Command hallucinations weren't a strong feature, we weren't concerned about him acting on command hallucinations while he was here, but he's almost certainly using more cannabis since he's been out of hospital and that's affecting his mental state."

James asked Mohinder whether he could bring up the CTO paperwork on the laptop he was using to type the minutes of the meeting. He wanted to gauge the conditions under which Manu could be returned to the ward. Then James asked Jean-Paul to invite Manu into the meeting. James turned to Abbie and quietly commented: "There's some things that you can't work with, like threats and knives." "Yeah, babies, hmm", Abbie responded. "To be honest you can't negotiate, you've got to admit", James said.

Manu entered the room and introductions were completed. James asked him how he had been. Manu was keen to emphasise how important for him it was to try to find a job. James acknowledged this, and then raised Aaron's concerns around the use of cannabis, the impact on Manu's finances and mental health and the voices telling him to kill people. Manu denied this. He said the voices were "just trying to put me down. They recognise that I've just come out of hospital, so they're just trying to get me back into hospital again. They want me out of there." Manu then returned to the issue of finding a job, explaining how this would benefit his mental health:

'I just have to be busy, keep occupied. It's the only way I can do this. I was going to go to the job centre today. I'm going to go after, after this meeting. I'll be distracted, it'd be different even from sitting in a room listening to voices. I'd be doing something.'

James argued that going straight into work may be taking things at too fast a pace, and he encouraged Manu to break this ambition down into intermediate steps towards his ultimate goal. James then returned to the topic of the "rules and boundaries" necessary for the Britchcombe Road staff to work safely with Manu and raised the issue of the knife found in his room. Manu could not remember how it got there. James said:

'There's a rule that sharp knives don't leave the kitchen, those kind of things. They found a sharp knife in your room and you've had hallucinations about killing a Ghanaian member of staff. That's a point where they can't work with you anymore. It's too risky. So we've got to talk about this and work out how can we, what can you do, what part can you play in making this work and, it seems to me it's difficult for you, it's a big change after being in hospital for a very long time. So what can we do to support you enough to make it work? That's the question.'

Manu said: "I don't think anyone can support me except for me making the choice myself. Plus I'm going to quit smoking then, I'm gonna do it. If I can't then there's a reason. If I can't I need it for a reason." "What's the reason?" James asked. Manu responded: "I don't need it, I don't need it, I'm trying to cut it out myself, I'm trying to cut it out myself."

In this exchange with Manu, James reframed the concern about risk into an exploration of the ways more institutional assistance could be made available. Manu's response was to reject the need for support. He considered the solution to reside at the individual level, in the mobilisation of his own personal resources. Manu's subsequent shift from a slightly ambivalent 'choice' position regarding cannabis use to a more unambiguous commitment to cutting out smoking seemed to signal his realisation of a further significant dimension: the context of institutional power that framed this interaction.

While the issue of power had remained implicit at that stage, it surfaced soon after. James explained his rationale for recommending drug treatment to Manu at length. But that seemed not to register with Manu, who returned to the topic of finding work. Then James issued a stark reminder:

'The other thing, of course, is that you are under a community treatment order and the conditions of a treatment order are that you work with the staff there, that's part of it. And, you know, not using drugs in the project, not spending all your money on drugs and trying to do things which are going to be good for your health.'

Then James negotiated. He raised the prospect of a change in the plan, involving a more phased transition to the hostel, with Manu returning to spend two or three nights a week in hospital. James said he thought Britchcombe Road was the environment best equipped to support Manu, but that it could be "jeopardised" by recent events:

'I think you have a will to do well, but it's been so long since you've had to take full responsibility. We recognise that, and we're not blaming you for it, but it's a fact. Maybe you have to take that responsibility more gradually and our support is very protective in some ways. I don't want to put you back into the full protection of hospital, that would be bad for you, but I want you to be able to take steps at the right kind of pace so you take responsibility for yourself and it feels alright rather than perhaps loading you with responsibility for yourself and it feeling difficult and you smoking a lot.'

In making the case for a balance between responsibility and protection, James framed his argument around the impact of institutionalisation on this service user's development in terms that were accessible for Manu. And he urged Manu to recognise the need for a slower pace of change towards greater responsibility. He reassured Manu that he was not to blame for this predicament, and suggested his increased use of cannabis could be associated with the additional pressures generated by the move into a hostel setting where there were lower levels of support than he had been used to.

James then went on to reinforce to Manu that he understood the "vicious circle" that sometimes develops when people who hear voices use cannabis to help them deal with the fear and paranoia associated with this experience. The problem, he explained, is that "the kickback from cannabis makes the voices and the paranoia worse".

Manu, however, did not agree with the proposal for a more phased transition. He was getting "loads of bad remarks, saying what are you doing in hospital. The more I'm in here the more I get depressed." His mother interjected to encourage him to accede to the plan. Manu turned towards her, raising his voice and speaking more rapidly. "I don't want to come back mum, you just want to see me, you're trying to get rid of me, you're trying to give me away. You've been doing that since I was a little baby, since I was five, you gave me away to grandma." She laughed nervously, then asked: "When, when?" Manu barely paused for breath and said:

'When people see that they start talking about why is the son in hospital, and you've got nothing to explain. Ah leave him he's a drug addict, he's a drug addict, hospital will do him good. Maybe he'll live there for the rest of his life. He's gonna need to stay there for 20 years in and out, 20 years. He's got no life.'

Manu then turned his attention towards the ward:

'Why don't the hospital just let me go, get on and do my own thing. Why won't the hospital just let me go, just let me do my own thing. I was good on my own. Why is everyone butting in, "You can't do that, you can't do that, you can't." I get that everywhere I go. "You can't do that, you can't do that, you can't come with us." If I can't do that, then just leave me alone to do my own thing. Let me go, go to work or something, I'm not a baby anymore. I'm tired of all this discipline stuff, man. You're getting on my back as well, my back's hurting because of all this.'

Manu stopped. James waited a few moments. He then asked gently what he thought the solution might be. Manu replied, at first with a sense of resignation:

'To get out, to get out of hospital. I don't wanna come back here anymore, I'll start getting names everywhere. Oh, look at Manu, he was nice when he was a child, oh look at him grown up to stay in hospital every year. People are talking about me every day. That's why I'm getting psychotic when people are talking about me every day.'

Manu's frustration escalated again:

'How many people saw me stop taking cannabis and then they give it to me, why do they do it? I stay away from them, then he comes back to me again, what are you doing around there, what are you doing, doing this, don't come to our house anymore, you start shouting … asking for £10, you're gonna buy cannabis, you're mutilating me, you're mutilating me, you don't wanna give me money, you don't wanna, you don't want me to be happy.'

I was looking at the floor while Manu was speaking. My eyes flicked up briefly. Everyone else was looking down or straight ahead. Occasionally they glanced across towards Manu but not for more than a moment. The exception was James. He looked steadily at Manu to show him he was listening.

Manu continued, distraught:

'It's about cannabis, it's not about me. Cannabis has got more respect than me. I'm not getting respect. The cannabis is getting respect. Every time the cannabis gets in my life that's it. On Sunday they're standing on the street and they're all shouting at me and everyone's watching me. "This druggy, he's supposed be goin' church on Sunday, he's not at church, he's got some money to buy cannabis." Everyone can hear that in the street. That causes problems. That really messes up my mental status.'

Then silence. The tense atmosphere pervading the room persisted. After a few moments more, James attempted to reassure Manu. "We're not against you. We want you to continue to do well, but you need more support." James then adjourned the meeting.

Manu and his mother left. The remaining practitioners glanced at each other with relief. The junior doctor commented: "He's psychotic." Abbie agreed: "Very psychotic, low mood, very angry." "He has to come back in", James concluded, before speculating on whether he might be inflaming the situation. "With mum here he can let it out", Abbie contended. "Actually he's upset with his family", added nurse Jean-Paul. James smiled back at

Jean-Paul and recounted that Manu had stopped making eye contact with him at one point, "so I backed off!"

Aaron asked if there was any way that drug and alcohol treatment conditions could be added to the CTO. James explained: "No. I think he's pre-contemplative. The psychological process of acting on not using drugs, he's a long way from that. The stage we're at is establishing boundaries, so let's avoid getting into a situation where we're nagging." James turned to Mohinder, and said: "I don't want to give a completely negative message that feeds into his shame. The forensic assessment suggested rehab. If he fails at Britchcombe Road then there's nowhere else but rehab."

James's perspective, part 1

As with Abbie, I interviewed James a year later, as I was completing the first phase of fieldwork, and asked him to reflect on his work with Manu.

Defining service user needs

James said:

> 'We were and he was faced with a kind of recurring situation in which he would get better, a little bit better in hospital and gain some independence from the hospital, go out, take drugs, get worse, lose his independence because of risk issues, become more psychotic and this cycle was going on for years. And, as far as I know, continues to this day.'

James thought Manu was caught in a "kind of intractable cycle of disability and I imagine, you know, a vicious circle of frustration and anger and dependence".
James explained:

> 'In some ways, Manu's actually a very dependent person and he's behaving in a way which is ensuring continuing detention, whether he's aware of it or not. And so he seems unable to, you know, be able to manage even a small amount of freedom from the hospital and because then he doesn't have the experience of learning how to manage it before the inevitable setback, he only ever reaches the same stage, so you know, it's like an elastic dependency, and he's very ill.'

James understood Manu's inability to successfully manage the transition in terms of problems rooted in his developmental learning process:

> 'He's gone from being a child to an adolescent with schizophrenia and so he'd never had the opportunity to develop an identity or any kind

of premorbid goals or sense of himself. He just didn't get anywhere near far enough to be thinking about, you know, higher-order things such as work and independence. He actually needed to achieve [a] reduction in symptoms and to experience that that was possible and to, just to experience some basic things. But I mean the dilemma there is it's not enough, it's not enough to, it wasn't enough to motivate him. And in the absence of anything more meaningful he would just repeatedly turn to drugs, that was his reward system. Do you see what I'm saying? So that almost because he hadn't had time to develop as a person as an adult, to develop other systems of reward you know, he was very restricted and he, he clearly got a bigger hit from crack cocaine than from, you know, just staying in hospital and not hearing such severe voices that's, that's too nebulous whereas the hit from crack cocaine is something he could relate to.'

After James had set out these dimensions of psychosis, substance misuse and dependency, I asked how he understood causality here. James said he had "an ideological bias towards social constructions, but we don't seem to have identified specific social events associated with schizophrenia". But he thought there was "something about human social organisation which is sufficient to trigger schizophrenia in biologically vulnerable individuals. Where do the proportions lie? I don't know."

James explained that he had ruled out family history, in the systemic rather than genetic sense. The family were, he later clarified, "close-knit" and although Manu's father displayed some "moral rigidity", for James this seemed to conform to Nigerian cultural norms. However, he was keen to emphasise that, in any case, he rejected a notion of schizophrenogenic families that labels and blames. He added: "I wouldn't say that I could identify factors in his life story that necessarily led to his condition, although probably they did." Consequently, James had "fallen back on a kind of, you know, biological construct for [Manu's] condition, so it was just a fact, he has this condition and it's caused severe disability".

While James evoked social processes, these were limited to the interpersonal level. His considerations (and those of the other practitioners) did not include the effects of structurally emergent features, for instance systemic, institutional and interpersonal racism. This will be discussed further at the end of the chapter.

Southville CMHT team meeting

At Southville, about one month after the ward rounds, the weekly team meeting was drawing to its close. Deputy team manager Filipe asked whether James had any other service users to discuss in the 'clinical' section of the meeting. "No", he replied, but then corrected himself and with a sigh continued, "oh, Manu …". James then brought the assembled practitioners up to date with developments, turning towards and addressing Abbie in particular:

> 'Manu's doing quite well, so he'd managed to go to Mayfield Walk [day centre] with the occupational therapist in the last week and the DDU [drug dependency unit], although he got angry and left. But now Britchcombe Road have said they don't want to keep him. I don't know if you're aware of that.'

James described his frustration with regard to an interaction between the Britchcombe Road manager and Manu that, for him, illustrated some of the reasons for the breakdown in the placement.

> 'The manager came last week to the ward round and I wasn't very impressed … She turned to talk to him, was nagging, negative, it was actually not the way to talk to a young adult with mental health problems and boundary issues, you know, because then you set up a systemic thing, where he's going to behave more like a teenager and rebel.'

However, James then went on to develop a systemic analysis that shifted the focus away from individual failures.[3]

> 'It's harder for them than for us, you know. It's not like a ward, where they've got lots of trained staff; they're a hostel, so it is harder and they're not as trained, but they just can't cope with it. You know, he's probably at least ten years younger than the next person in the place. It's the people who have been through the forensic system and they're all quite kind of institutionalised.'

James explained that Manu needed a more 'nurturing' environment than Britchcombe Road offered. "It's basic stuff with people with schizophrenia, you don't just give them criticism, negative feedback." James described his attempts to model a more appropriate approach but, despite this, the Britchcombe manager persisted with an "all guns blazing" attitude towards Manu:

> 'I'd kind of set the scene by saying [to Manu]: "These are the positive aims and these are the boundaries that, you know, the expectations that we all would have of you as well", as a negotiation … But then she started talking, she was really: "You haven't been doing this, you haven't been doing that, you've got to do this."'

Abbie's response to this news indicated she did not share James's perspective. There were growing tensions. She said:

'I have to say, I'm not completely surprised, I always found his behaviour in that hostel really, really, really disturbed and you could see from the top that the people that I met in the ward rounds were very concerned. It was a prevailing attitude at every single meeting and we're very, you know, we're concerned with him and there was no break to that and I think we did really well trying to encourage them and trying to support them and tried to explain that behaviour, saying, you know: "It's a different move for him, he's got to settle, it's a very difficult, you know, transition for him." But I am not surprised, because I always found his behaviour disturbing.'

James replied:

'He's going to be difficult to place anywhere, isn't he? They're the same kind of concerns but, you know, we'd responded to that by slowing it down and having him back in hospital and there hadn't been any new kind of knife-type issues or, you know, which they were still referring back to that, which was stretching back weeks and weeks. So I think they hadn't, they'd kind of taken hold of a particular point of view and so I'm, at the moment, I don't know where we're going to.'

James located the problem at the systemic level, with the breakdown of the placement triggered by a communication problem within the social system at Britchcombe Road. Although he recognised the limitations on Britchcombe Road as a result of the institutionalisation experiences of service users there and the lower skill levels among staff, James identified the dominant problem as the rigid and authoritarian style of interaction with Manu. This instituted a negative feedback loop that reproduced homeostasis and prevented positive change.

Although Abbie did not directly challenge this analysis, she wanted to refocus on the individual level of Manu's 'disturbing' behaviour. Other team members at the meeting began to suggest other possible accommodation options for Manu. But Abbie was keen to return to the risk posed by Manu. This debate revealed more starkly the contrasting views. Abbie continued:

'The thing about Manu that really intrigues me is that he registered with that GP really quickly, so he kind of resettled, but never settled. You know there was a real contradiction in his behaviour and he never turned up for any of the meetings with them. But I always did feel that he was really paranoid and dangerous.'

"Yeah, he is," James said. "He is dangerous, but he hasn't *been* that dangerous yet. I mean the risk assessment is scary, as in terms of potential." Abbie replied: "But his behaviour in the hostel, you know, continually having a knife in his room, threatening a pregnant worker, lots and lots of instances, one after the other, after the other." James said: "Yeah, but he didn't threaten anybody with the knife, he had the knife in his room, so". "But he talked about it," Abbie said. "Well no," James responded, "he talked about having auditory hallucinations about a member of staff. But, I don't know, if he's too dangerous for somewhere like that, then he's too dangerous for anywhere. That's, you know, that's the place where they're resourced to be able to do risk assessments."

This illustrated a pattern. James consistently challenged the labelling of Manu by team members or practitioners from other services. For instance, at a team meeting several months earlier, Bill, a community mental health nurse (CMHN), had referred to Manu and another service user with whom he had had an altercation as "dangerous people". James had looked exasperated and disputed this, saying that he did not think Manu was the most dangerous of people, and reminding Bill that the team works with lots of potentially dangerous people.

James's perspective, part 2

During my interview with James a year later, he was still frustrated at the team's failure to help Manu.

Strategies for intervention

At the first ward round, James had described a 'medication, boundaries and encouragement' strategy. Critically reflecting back on this approach, he focused mainly on the latter two:

> 'On the one hand, we were doing the same thing again and again, so I guess responding in an institutional way or institutionalised way, making sure that he and other people were as safe as possible, you know, reducing his access to drugs when he was unwell by reducing his freedom. And then at the same time, a parallel process of desperately trying to think how to do things differently, how to create a different outcome. How to help him to think about himself in a different way, whether that was through just talking or through trying to engage him in, you know, through occupational therapy etcetera, in other forms of activity than drug taking, so stimulation or helping him make friends or have more positive relationships, whilst being institutionalised in hospital.'

Here, 'boundaries' is rearticulated as a custodial 'institutionalisation' strategy that serves to manage risk by restricting Manu's liberty and thus reducing his access to drugs. Similarly, 'encouragement' is reframed as forms of talking and occupational therapy aiming to improve Manu's engagement, social functioning and emotional development, and to assist him to achieve a more positive self-conception by promoting new ways of thinking about himself. This second strand evokes a social-relational approach.

James described the combination of these two components as an institutionally defined strategy to create a "protective bubble" and minimise the potential for harm so that Manu "stands a better chance of surviving, just not dying through, you know, involvement in the drugs scene and violence that kind of thing. And also he's receiving active treatment through medication for his condition and so is at lower risk of ... the cognitive deterioration of schizophrenia." Thus, for James, the purpose of institutionalisation was to reduce risks *to* Manu from a violent drug scene and from cognitive decline purportedly arising from non-treatment with antipsychotic medication.

James continued by articulating these significant tensions between the two parallel strands of custodial institutionalisation and therapy:

'So, you know, these were kind of opposite processes in some way, clearly both necessary. But the side effect of the institutionalisation, which we could see, we were aware of, seemed to be making him more dependent and less able to cope with any form of independence or self-management, if you like. And so we had to somehow undo that process ourselves, you know, through a parallel of trying to give him freedom and responsibility. Anyway, it didn't work and he's still there.'

This passage reveals James's frustration at the failure of this strategy and acknowledges the contradiction that lay at the heart of it. Both strands were perceived as necessary, but the work of the first functioned to 'undo' the effects of the second. In this way, institutionalised risk management presented an obstacle to therapeutic success. This highlights the tension and incompatibility between social-relational (therapeutic) approaches and custodial interventions.

In the interviews, James said relatively little about the third strand of his strategy: medication. Nonetheless, the discussions from the first ward round highlighted the centrality of Manu's adherence to the medication treatment plan. Without this it would be 'quickly' deemed necessary to recall him to the ward. This suggests that the risk to be managed by medication was not only to Manu, as James noted, but also from him.

Making professional judgements: systemic thinking and biopsychosocial psychiatry

At the beginning of the interview, James explained that, while initially interested in psychotherapy during his training, he soon found this to be too narrow in focus. He came to prefer the variety and intensity of general psychiatry, because "you're dealing with real, you know, severe hardship and social deprivation". In particular, he identified with working in a "holistic way, it wasn't just medication, it's not just therapy but I suppose biopsychosocial psychiatry, in all its fullness".

This holistic approach was discernible in James's use of systemic frameworks for understanding Manu's experiences. This was illustrated by his description of the attempt to discharge Manu from the inpatient ward to the Britchcombe Road.

'I think it was pretty much a failure all round. I don't think [Britchcombe Road] had the opportunity to work with him fully. I don't think [Manu] gave them the opportunity, but I think they didn't take what was offered either and it was quite disappointing. They talked about him in very negative terms and I think, I don't know, it just seemed, you know, if you think about it in systemic terms, that we were all caught up in this repeating cycle and that even, you know, professional groupings who were only lately brought into it, like the Britchcombe Road team, very quickly were kind of co-opted into this particular narrative of failure and relapse and risk and you know, the inevitability of it all. It seemed to be that, on some level, [that] is what was going on inside Manu.'

Here the breakdown in the relationship between Manu and the staff at the hostel was evident in the failure of either party to grasp the opportunity to engage in therapeutic work. However, this failure developed in a context of the negative labelling of Manu. This generated a self-fulfilling prophecy in the form of a narrative of inevitable failure, which was then internalised by Manu. This orientation evokes 'soft' labelling (Link and Phelan, 1999), where this social process is understood to exacerbate the effects, rather than constitute the cause, of mental distress.

In a systemic sense, then, the problems in the placement of Manu and his behavioural dependency became an emergent feature of the social and institutional system within which he found himself. James thus extended the locus of responsibility beyond the individual, locating an understanding of the problems in an organisational context rather than within the service user himself.

One consequence of this systemic failure was the difficulty in supporting Manu to generate any idea of what his recovery might look like in view of the impacts of his condition on his development. For James, it felt like "giving up. It's quite pessimistic, which was, you know, emotionally difficult really working with a very young man. It felt like condemning him to more of the same for the next few years, you know, the best years of his youth."

The way in which Manu presented also generated a form of misrecognition of his needs that fed into the negative institutional cycle:

> 'We work with a lot of people who are very severely disabled with schizophrenia and severe chronic negative symptoms and cognitive symptoms. And he didn't seem to have that. His personality appeared to be underdeveloped but intact and, you know, his, his cognition seemed to be intact so perhaps, you know, for professionals because there wasn't such a visible disability that added to the frustration and perhaps the mistake in having expectations which were too high in the present. And we should have had expectations about a different rate of change, a slower rate of change, and that as a result he just kept failing and failing and failing, which reinforced the idea that failure was inevitable.'

While James noted earlier that the goal of the work was to support Manu to overcome dependence in order to achieve freedom, independence and self-management, he indicated here a pressure from professionals for this service user to take on a level of responsibility that James saw as unrealistic at that moment.

This was underpinned by James's broader critical appraisal of discourses such as *individual responsibilisation*. He advocated instead a 'sick role' position. This brings into view philosophical questions of the extent to which responsibility for actions should reside solely with the individual experiencing mental distress. Those advocating the sick role have frequently looked to an organic model to support the position that the person should not be held responsible, while a moral model has been articulated by those who believe the individual should be held primarily accountable (Miresco and Kirmayer, 2006). However, while the sick role concept tends to be associated with medical paternalism, James articulated his perspective in terms of a rejection of contemporary neoliberal sociopolitical transformations: "I hate it when patients are called customers. It just seems a lie as if they have the choice and the rights of a customer, that they're consuming something ... by calling somebody a customer you somehow cheat them out of their sick role." James linked the undermining of the sick role with the development of a consumerist orientation towards service users. He went on to clarify this:

> 'It justifies not providing care. Look it's, it's, it's complex you know, because on the one hand it's as, as, a service ideology and

structure which encourages people to be, towards autonomy is good, autonomy is good, patient autonomy is good. But along a spectrum if that's taken too far and the patient then is deemed to have total responsibility for their behaviour and, so it's a kind of Thomas Szasz model, so if they commit a crime they should go to prison, you know, if they swear at a hostel worker they should be evicted, then I think that's highly problematic and then they're not being allowed their sick role. So not only, you know, could it be argued that they've been unfortunate enough to have this condition, not only in general does society shit on them through stigma and through exclusion, now they're not allowed the care which would have been the compensation from society, the meagre compensation for that. They're called customers and they're expected to control themselves when, by definition, part of having a mental illness is sometimes you lose control, not always, but it's necessary to have a dynamic changing idea of when somebody can and when they can't be autonomous ... And some people may say that's paternalistic but I think it's realistic.'

The erosion of the sick role is thus linked with the emergence of neoliberalism, enacted through the extension of the market and consumerism into the mental health service domain. For James, these broader systemic pressures and associated demands for Manu to reach markers of self-management and responsibilisation too rapidly contributed to the narrative of failure surrounding this service user.

Abbie's perspective, part 2

In her interview at about the same time, Abbie took a more positive view of what was happening with Manu. He was now a patient on a psychiatric intensive care unit (PICU) and had been referred to a 'low secure' forensic inpatient setting.

Strategies for intervention

Abbie explained: "He's now on Lyneham PICU, which is absolutely superb. Love going there, love the staff, just I'm just so behind that kind of, when it's really needed, you treat, you treat the behaviour, you treat the illness." This was a dual-pronged strategy where behaviour, rooted in personality, was treated alongside Manu's 'psychotic illness'. However, the treatment of behaviour appeared to be a much higher priority for Abbie. PICUs form a bridge between general psychiatric and 'low secure' forensic inpatient settings, offering more 'intensive' forms of intervention.

'It's all locked. But, honestly, it might sound draconian, but he needs that. He needs the boundaries of someone saying: "No, you can't do that." I think he got away with his behaviour for so long, because he intimidates his family. He intimidates his Mum and his Dad just doesn't want to know. Dad just wants to get on with being a pastor and hopefully, you know, he'll get better, sort of thing. But he's a very big, strong boy and he would scare me. If I had to live with him, I'd be frightened of him.'

Abbie then went on to articulate the importance of a 'stricter' regime of boundaries:

'Low-secure boundaries, brilliant and that's what he needs. He's a young man and he needs, you know, he's kind of regressed to being a really nutty three- to four-year-old. I know my son would be like that if I let him, but we don't let him, you see. So that's about holding, holding, holding. It's so tough, especially with boys. [Her son] Billy would be a nutcase if I let him, you know, he'd just like hit and punch. But it's all boundaries, talk[ing] about "no" and setting bans on things and stuff like that and my guess is [whispers] Manu never had them.'

Here, Manu's family were constructed as both victims of Manu's aggression but also responsible for it. This perception was reinforced by their apparent unwillingness to take responsibility and engage with therapy. Abbie described setting up a family therapy meeting but "they didn't come. Nothing, didn't come and that tells me a lot about who's not in the room."

Ultimately Abbie's intention was for Manu to develop insight into his condition and behaviour. She regarded the pathway from PICU to a 'low secure' setting as a crucial means to do so:

'I've worked with a lot of male service users [who've] been through the forensic wards and they say: "Oh, they're brilliant, they're really good. The nurses understand what the problem is, they know how to help you, you get the rehab, you get the psychology and it's much stricter and it was what I needed." It's mainly that the staff understand it, that was the main thing that they've identified, so that's what I hope to bring to Manu.'

In this account Abbie evoked service users who had, with hindsight, recognised the benefits of this 'stricter' forensic environment. The perspective of these service users was highlighted several times by Abbie as a rationale for Manu's referral to low secure services. Another was that a wider range of services would be available to him in this setting. Access to such specialist interventions was thus offered as a key justification for more 'draconian' option.

Making professional judgements: the role of practical knowledge

Another significant dimension of Abbie's decision making was the relationship between 'knowing' and 'experience', described by her in the process of developing understanding of Manu's needs.

> 'I'd say, you know, we're going to go for a low secure forensic unit. I mean, that was me doing the risk assessments and looking at this list and just, this boy's forensic and that was experience, just knowing, this is not a section 3 [of MHA] going to a hostel, this is more, this is worse.'

Trial and error over a long period of practice enabled Abbie to learn to trust her 'gut feeling':

> 'Years and years and years of doing, of not listening to it, doing stuff, doing stuff which was logical or not doing what I felt, just doing something else. And then thinking, don't, I wish I'd gone with my gut feeling or what was in my heart. So years of sort of getting it wrong and then eventually just, you know, [laughs] just, you know, it's right, 'cause you feel it.'

What Abbie was evoking in these passages were forms of practical knowledge. Such tacit forms of knowing are embodied as skilful dispositions, a 'feel for the game' developed through experience in this field over many years (Bourdieu, 1977). However, while Abbie had practised as a nurse within inpatient and day hospital settings for more than 20 years, she was new to community work, having only worked in the CMHT for just over a year. The ward and hospital are institutionalised contexts in which risk management is given high priority. The tacit forms of knowledge Abbie had developed in this environment seemed to be shaping her conceptions of the work with Manu in more risk-averse ways.

The contrast between theoretical and practical knowledge was also apparent in Abbie's comment, later in the interview, that: "I'm not romantic or I haven't got great theories or big ideas about things. I'm very boring, down to earth." Abbie somewhat apologetically contrasted her practical approach with both medically oriented diagnostic practices and technical skills for therapeutic intervention, as Chapter 3 noted. "I haven't got anything else," she said. "I mean, I've done a CBT [cognitive behavioural therapy] course and I think I remember one dynamic question from it ... I've done a counselling course and I can just about remember to sort of repeat what they said." She laughed and went on:

> 'I've done, you know, different courses and different things, but I don't have, some people have got a skill box, you know and they're like: "I

can use this approach and that approach" and this is where I feel, God, I'm so inadequate, because I don't have anything like that, I'm just me.'

'Race', racism and situational logics

The mental health system responses to Manu's lived experiences were primarily framed by a focus on risk management. Consequently, particular emergent institutional features of the setting were foregrounded by James, Abbie and others. The first was a *discourse of danger and violence*, a prominent lens through which this service user was perceived. Restrictions on Manu's autonomy were then justified through a second feature: paternalism *(medical dominance)*. Attendant organisational responses were based on management through institutionalisation *(custodialism)* and medication *(biomedical model)*. These four emergent features combined to to form a 'situational logic' that was widely visible during the fieldwork in relation to service users who were perceived to be moving into a 'crisis' phase. This logic generated an institutional (or, in EM, 'directional') tendency towards what I call 'custodial paternalism'.

However, while the reflections on Manu's needs by James, Abbie and other practitioners included a range of causal factors and strategies for intervention, there was a significant omission. These explorations of this service user's lived experiences did not explicitly consider what role may have been played by racism and mental distress processes of racialisation.

People from racialised groups, and African and Caribbean young men in particular, experience multiple structural and institutional disadvantages linked to racial discrimination, such as higher rates of unemployment, poorer housing and over-representation in the criminal justice system (Keating, 2007). These structural inequalities combine with cumulative exposure to everyday racism to increase levels of mental distress (Wallace et al, 2016). Structural, institutional and interpersonal racism also produces racialised inequalities within the mental health system (Nazroo et al, 2020). Pathways into services are marked by significant racial disparities, with Black or Black British people four times more likely than White people to be detained under the MHA (NHS Digital, 2021), eight times more likely to be subject to CTOs (Barkhuizen et al, 2020) and three times more likely to be given the diagnostic label of schizophrenia and admitted to hospital (Bignall et al, 2019). Having faced greater compulsion and coercion at their point of entry to services (Nazroo et al, 2020), people from racialised groups then experience more restricted access to social and psychological forms of support within this setting (McKenzie et al, 2001).

A prominent example of the interweaving of everyday racial bias with structural and institutional racism in the mental health system is the 'risk agenda' that emerged in the 1990s. Longstanding public conceptions of madness as 'alien' and 'violent' were amplified by a racialised dimension during this period because of policy and media representations of two prominent homicide cases involving people known to mental health services where the perpetrators were Black and the victims White (Butler and Drakeford, 2003).[4] Keating (2007) has noted the subsequent emergence of a stereotype of Black men as impulsive and dangerous,[5] and how such perceptions have combined with cultural ignorance and stigma to shape restrictive and punitive mental health service responses to people from racialised communities. However, this is reinforced by a much longer history of the racialisation of mental distress, which continues to permeate contemporary psychiatry and mental health services. This refers to the legacy of the interleaving of eugenic concepts associated with racialised hierarchies[6] and theories of biomedical causation within psychiatry's knowledge base during its formative years in the early 20th century (Pilgrim, 2008; Harrison, and Burke, 2020).

Understanding the absence of these powerful dynamics of racial discrimination from practitioners' reflections on Manu's experiences is critical. The notion of situational logics and strategic directional tendencies within EM enables a focus that acknowledges, but also extends beyond, individual-level biases and discriminatory attitudes. In doing so, EM provides a framework for understanding the way in which systemic processes and institutional tendencies shape dominant practices and ideas to produce such omissions. A starting point for this is recognition of how processes of racialisation and colonialism are integral to many of the emergent features of neoliberal mental health services, and consequently underpin dominant situational logics and directional tendencies such as custodial paternalism and biomedical residualism. The *biomedical model*, is a key feature of both these directional tendencies and, as noted above, its genesis was informed by eugenic ideas of racial hierarchy. Similarly, the *discourse of danger and violence* associated with extreme forms of distress has been powerfully shaped, in both its historic and contemporary manifestations, by the ideology of structural racism. Moreover, as a consequence of the latter discourses, *informational practice systems* oriented to risk management and prudentialism tend to generate situated forms of knowledge that embed racialised perceptions of risk (Nazroo et al, 2020). Finally, in foregrounding individual-level and biodeterministic constructions of service user *responsibilisation,* a dominant psychocentric orientation under neoliberalism de-emphasises structural and institutional-level causal accounts of mental distress.

As these elements combine to form dominant situational logics in contemporary mental health services, they shape the ideational and practical horizons of mental health workers through directional tendencies such as custodial paternalism and biomedical residualism. These dominant logics and tendencies thus marginalise considerations on the role of racialised inequalities (as well as other structural dynamics) in causing and exacerbating mental distress, and thereby reinforce gaps and silences on 'race' and racism. This enables further institutionalisation of racism within service interventions regardless of the intentions of individual practitioners.[7] In James's view, mental health services had failed Manu. The notion of situational logics and directional tendencies offers a lens for understanding why.

5

Defining mental distress

This second individual case study chapter discusses the interventions of workers from Southville Community Mental Health Team (CMHT) and the local mental health inpatient unit with a service user, Alistair, and his wife and informal carer, Felicity. I explore the different constructions of Alistair's mental health needs elaborated by Dr James Bryant, his consultant psychiatrist, Filipe, his care coordinator/social worker, Felicity and Alistair himself. The implications of transitions between 'stable' and 'acute' phases for the way in which practitioners understand and respond to this service user's experiences of mental distress are also explored.

Alistair

Alistair is a 44-year-old White British man, who holds a senior management post in a large international insurance firm. Alistair's first contact with secondary mental health services was two years ago. He was initially treated in the private sector, paid for by his employer, but was subsequently transferred to care in the National Health Service (NHS). He has had three admissions to NHS psychiatric inpatient units during this period, one of which was elective to begin treatment with medication. Alistair was given the diagnostic label of bipolar affective disorder. He was married to Felicity, and they had three children. Although Alistair and Felicity had recently separated, she was still heavily involved in providing support to him and acted as an informal carer. Felicity regularly attended the Trust's carers' support group.

Treatment and intervention

This section provides an overview of how James, Filipe and ward staff developed their understandings of Alistair's mental health needs.

James summarised his view of the development of Alistair's mental health needs in a letter to his general practitioner (GP). The letter was written after James first saw Alistair for an outpatient appointment following an admission to an inpatient psychiatric unit during the preceding summer.

> He has had instability of mood since March [last year]. This started with a manic episode with psychotic symptoms, for example he believed his colleague was a secret service agent involved in a plot to kill his wife.

He was also experiencing auditory hallucinations in the form of beeps and whistles, which at the time he believed underlined and emphasised certain things that have been said. He also believed he was Jesus. The severe elevation of his mood lasted approximately four weeks, although as time progressed he became less psychotic. ... Around mid-May his mood changed and he became depressed.

James noted that Alistair had 'now had in total four or five hypomanic or manic episodes with psychotic symptoms and one depressive episode. Technically he fulfils criteria for bipolar affective disorde'.

However, James acknowledged that Alistair did not agree with the diagnosis, explaining that he 'was very stigmatised by this'. James's response was to encourage 'him to think about his mental health problems not in terms of labels, but rather a problem-solving approach, in order to generate potential solutions'. This is evocative of Healy (2008), who notes a convergence towards a more United States-style consumerist orientation in psychiatry in the United Kingdom where practitioners are now increasingly expected to become enablers of problem solving by patients rather than experts in their more traditional role in treating disease entities. James concluded: 'In my opinion, he is more likely to benefit from a mood stabiliser than an antipsychotic and he agreed to consider a trial of Lithium Carbonate.'

In a further letter to the GP, James noted that following an earlier episode of treatment in the private sector, funded by his employer, Alistair 'apparently ... briefly became elevated again in response to being prescribed Citalopram 40mg. This was subsequently withdrawn.' In a later summary of Alistair's treatment, James explained that this service user was admitted to the Upton Ward at the Middletown Centre inpatient unit to commence lithium carbonate. However, Alistair 'was also prescribed an antidepressant – citalopram – and an antipsychotic – olanzapine. The purpose of the antipsychotic was to reduce the risk that the antidepressant would trigger an iatrogenic[1] manic episode'.

This polypharmaceutical approach should be understood in the context of the increased emphasis on risk management. In Alistair's case, this took the form of suicide risk, an issue raised in James's next letter to the GP. In September of that year, Alistair's wife had discovered in his diary a 'suicide plan to kill himself with carbon monoxide poisoning'. Alistair was admitted again to inpatient care shortly after. Healy (2006) notes that the perceived high risk of suicide among those diagnosed with type 1 bipolar disorder creates a significant pressure for doctors to treat this population with psychotropic medication.[2]

Around this time, Alistair was also offered a place at the local mental health day hospital, 'which would have provided a higher level of support, monitoring and therapy on his discharge from the inpatient unit'. However, James noted that Alistair declined this service.

> He is quite set on wanting to continue to go to work on a part-time basis. I am concerned that his poor performance at work will reinforce his depression and anxiety and hinder his recovery. We have discussed this at length with Alistair and his wife and we will have to monitor the effect this may have on his mental state.

James's attitude was consistent with his advocacy of the 'sick role', described in Chapter 4.

ART meeting with Filipe and 'step down'

At this stage Filipe, deputy manager and social worker, became involved in providing some short-term support to Alistair. This was via the Acute Response Team[3] (ART) within the CMHT, with an expectation to provide short-term transitional support as Alistair transferred to the outpatient clinic. When I asked Filipe if he and James conducted ART meetings with Alistair jointly, Filipe shook his head and told me they worked separately, explaining that James provided "the medical model", while he offered "psychological treatment". With Alistair and Filipe's consent, I was able to join one of the ART meetings.

As we walked back to Filipe's office after the meeting, I asked him about James's referral of Alistair to the Trust's psychology department for cognitive-behavioural therapy (CBT), which had been mentioned at the meeting. Filipe lowered his voice slightly, explaining that he thought that many of the team's clients needed therapy, and yet Alistair "seems to have gone ahead in the queue". He expressed surprise that Alistair had been seen so quickly and by Spencer, Head of Psychology. He then hinted that perhaps James had arranged this for him directly with the psychology department but asked me not to disclose this view. Filipe went on to describe Alistair's senior project management role in the insurance sector. Although he did not explicitly causally link these two issues, my interpretation was that Filipe was suggesting that Alistair's status and social class background may have been a factor in the apparent 'preferential treatment' that facilitated his swift access to this service.

Filipe then turned to his computer, apparently wanting to start his notes for RiO. He wrote:

> Alistair was seen today. He reported that he saw James on 20th January and has reduced his olanzapine, however he continues to take lithium and citalopram which find them helpful and no side affects [sic]. He is still feeling a bit sleepy during the afternoon and in the evening.

He has no problems with sleeping and appetite. His concentration has improved. He saw a clinical psychologist, Spencer last week for an assessment and he will see him again next week to start CBT – i.e. to help him with prioritising his work. He will see his Occupational Health Officer within 3 weeks to discuss possibility to return to full time work. At present he is working 4 days a week (Wednesday is off). He has agreed to stop session with me, however I reassured him that he can contact me before 11th March (next outpatient appointment) if there is a need to do so. Plan – Stepdown to see James in his [outpatient] clinic and attend sessions with psychologist. Case closed to me.

One of the most notable features is that, while questions around medication and biological symptoms were relatively briefly addressed in the session itself, they were accorded a higher priority within this written account. The pressure to monitor and record biomedical indicators reflects the prominence of 'chemical imbalance' theories of mental illness within services. The aetiology of conditions such as depression has long been linked by mainstream psychiatry with a deficit of the neurotransmitter serotonin, associated with the regulation of appetite, sleep and emotion (Lacasse and Leo, 2005).[4] Consequently, checking biological indicators has become an integral element of institutional risk management regimes, requiring practitioners both to assess variations in patterns of sleep and appetite as possible symptoms of depression or other related mental health conditions and to monitor service users' medication 'compliance' (Ramon, 2005).

This mode of biomedical monitoring during the 'stable phase' is thus oriented to assessing and reinforcing responsible forms of conduct around medication by service users as part of wider risk management strategies that include prominent electronic record-keeping (informational) requirements.[5] Filipe's efforts to minimise this 'biomedical residualist' mode of practice in the meeting but its foregrounding in the recorded account indicated both resistance and reluctant acquiescence to this institutional tendency, which was in tension with his own professional and personal values. This has parallels with the reservations articulated by team manager Evelyn in Chapter 2, when she spoke somewhat disparagingly of these increasingly ubiquitous "sleep, mood and meds" questions and the monitoring practices associated with them.

Another salient contrast apparent in this scenario is that while issues around both work and family pressures were identified by Filipe as factors in the aetiology of Alistair's mental distress and explored at length in the meeting, only the former was recorded in the progress notes. This reflects the increasing priority accorded to seeking and maintaining employment within neoliberal active welfare regimes (Jessop, 1999). CBT, in particular, is considered an important facilitator of re-entry to the labour market

(Layard, 2005), in contrast to the more marginal status of systemic and psychosocial considerations.

James's account of Alistair's relapse and care coordinator allocation

Eight months after his step down to outpatients, Alistair was admitted to one of the wards at the Middletown Centre following a Mental Health Act (MHA) assessment. The Crisis Resolution Team had been working with him in the days leading up to this, but then felt 'he could no longer be managed at home'. As the ward's summary went on to explain, Alistair had 'reportedly reduced his dose of lithium of his own accord to 800mg and had become increasingly manic' during the two weeks before admission. James reiterated this perceived reason for the relapse in a subsequent letter to Alistair's employer's occupational health doctor:

> The most likely trigger for the manic episode is that Alistair reduced the dose of Lithium Carbonate. He did this as he had been feeling stable and most likely didn't realise that this reduction would have taken the Lithium level to a sub-therapeutic level. Lithium Carbonate is a maintenance medication taken to reduce the risk of relapse. Having reduced the dose of Lithium Carbonate he was then more vulnerable to experiencing a destabilisation of his mood.

Following this brief admission, Alistair was supported by the Crisis Resolution Team for two months, at which point his care was transferred to Southville CMHT and Filipe was allocated as his care coordinator.

Filipe and James's accounts of Alistair's eventual recovery

Over the next three months, Filipe monitored Alistair's mental state, which he described as stable. He gradually reduced the frequency of contact with Alistair, although also began to meet him together with Felicity. Filipe recorded in his notes that he discussed:

> the support needed for both of them as a couple. Felicity expressed her fears/anxiety about Alistair's mental illness. Discussed what happened prior to his last hospital admission ... There are many issues regarding their relationship and their children – Felicity described how it has been difficult for the children as they fear Alistair becoming ill again in the future.

This demonstrated a more systemic orientation. While Filipe did note that Alistair had restarted on a citalopram prescription during the previous week, he remained primarily oriented to social support, recording that this service user was facing the particular stressor of moving to his own flat (as Felicity and Alistair had agreed to live separately) while they worked on marital counselling.

For James, the key issue remained the impact of the reinstated treatment with citalopram. By July of that year, he recorded the following in Alistair's notes: 'There has been a great improvement in his mood since the increase in citalopram to 20mg. No sign of hypomania. Felicity reports a big improvement, saying he's much more engaged with other people.' Similarly, James noted in a letter to the GP:

I am pleased to say that overall, his insight has greatly improved and that this is likely to have a positive effect on his prognosis. The most likely trigger for the manic episode was that he took it upon himself to reduce the dose of Lithium without consultation and it is possible that this fell beneath therapeutic levels. I will see him again in a month.

In a letter to the occupational health department of Alistair's employer, James wrote:

Alistair and his care team have taken measures to reduce the risk and these involve changes in his medication, an increased level of community support and perhaps most importantly the learning experience that Alistair has gained and which will contribute to his ability to maintain his mental health in the future.

This emphasises the issue of responsibilisation and the management of risk, which is increasingly devolved to the service user. But this is within the parameters of professional knowledge, as demonstrated by Alistair's 'learning experience' from reducing his lithium to a sub-therapeutic level.

Conceptualising and responding to mental distress

This section will provide an overview of ways in which Alistair's experiences were conceptualised by members of the team and Alistair and Felicity, and their preferred approaches to support and intervention.

James's perspective

James began by describing Alistair, in diagnostic terms, as someone with "bipolar affective disorder – quite an unusual form of bipolar affective". The reason he considered Alistair's experiences to be atypical was that "he has very long phases of depression or mania, hypomania, and takes a long time to recover". Alistair had "had bipolar, a mild form of bipolar, for a long time. But the current pattern seems only to have started in the last two or three years". While James thus implicitly acknowledged that the onset of the condition in Alistair's 40s was, by the standards of the dominant biomedical framework, relatively late, this was rationalised as the intensification of a pre-existing but milder form of the condition.

James went on to explore the contextual and contributory factors leading to the development of Alistair's mental health issues. The two main factors he identified were work stress/dissonance and the constraints placed on him by his lifestyle and financial commitments. In relation to the first, James noted that Alistair was "a very intelligent man in some ways, so he has a highly paid job in the insurance world. But I don't think he's ever been happy in that job." He contrasted Alistair, a "gentle" and "thoughtful" man, with his work role "in the cut-throat world of finance". Consequently, as a result of "either the stress of work or the dissonance of working in an environment with people he doesn't identify with", he became "extremely anxious ... It just got too much for him". And Alistair also felt "trapped" by a high salary to cover a mortgage and a lifestyle that his family has become accustomed to.

However, having discussed environmental factors such as stress, James then considered the possible role of family relationships:

'Whether I was talking about biological aetiology, the family history of schizophrenia or the experience of growing up having close family relationships with people with major mental illness and the effect that has on your own development and your own ability to relate to other people. So, I think it's his mother who has schizophrenia, or brother, first degree relative with schizophrenia, possibly two, modelling a particular style of relating. And I think they are older siblings as well. So as well as the genetic, perhaps inherited risk, or changes in personality, it does seem from what his wife said that he has always been, this has always been a part of his character aside from changes that happened after he developed mood disorder.'

Thus, James rejected a straightforward reduction of the aetiology of Alistair's mental distress to either a singular biological or social causal process. Instead, he retained an open position in which both genetic inheritance and this service user's childhood sociodevelopmental environment may have played a role or interacted.

James noted that Alistair received a high level of input from services. He offered a clear rationale for this intensive input, stating: "I worry about the risk of suicide." This concern had emerged when Felicity had discovered an entry in Alistair's diary describing suicidal thoughts, which James described as a "vague suicide plan". A particular concern for James was that Alistair had not disclosed this to anyone, and "now he's not with his wife so he is not so closely monitored".

Strategies for intervention: the acute and stable phases

James noted that when deciding on or recommending strategies for intervention, the approach chosen "depends on the acuteness of the situation". James explained:

> 'So now I suppose we are thinking about relapse prevention and risk factors and early warning signs and advance directives and things like that, whereas eight, nine months ago we were thinking about things like lowering [Alistair's] mood, moderating the excesses of his disinhibited behaviour, supporting his wife through his acute episode and then helping negotiate with his employer to go back to work, so it just shifts depending on where he is in the cycle.'

James drew a contrast between two stages. At the 'acute phase' of the cycle, strategies included the use of medication to manage Alistair's mood, increased community and social support to Alistair and his wife and consideration of inpatient admission to monitor suicide risk and reduce other risks associated with 'disinhibited behaviour'. Meanwhile, during the 'stable phase', the focus was relapse prevention through the identification, prediction and management of longer-term risk. One technique suggested by James for achieving this was the advance directive. James illustrated its potential utility when describing a problematic early discharge several months earlier. Alistair, he explained, had presented as 'too well' and as a result was discharged prematurely from inpatient care by the psychiatrist responsible. This led to a "protracted manic episode" in the community, which was "very destructive for his family".

To avoid a reoccurrence of this, James had recommended Alistair and Filipe work on writing a letter or advance directive. James suggested the content should include an acknowledgement from Alistair that he was likely to request to leave hospital, that he "can affect the appearance of being relatively well when this isn't the case" and that early discharge might lead to serious consequences. James noted:

> 'If Alistair were to write this himself, partly for him to read if he's not that unwell, this might convince him to, this is a message from himself, but also for hospital staff to read and also potentially it, to be presented to an appeal tribunal, so if he is appealing actually, he could effectively be testifying against himself.'

While a number of audiences for this letter were identified, including inpatient practitioners and Mental Health Review Tribunal[6] members, a central target was Alistair himself. This demonstrates the extent to which contemporary services are oriented to supporting users to develop self-management strategies that are integrated within the broader requirements of services. Thus, service users are positioned as consumers as well as co-opted producers of services, reflecting both responsibilisation and paternalism (Gilliat et al, 2000).

Alistair's perspective

Alistair labelled his mental distress utilising the diagnostic category 'type 1 bipolar disorder' and described this experience in terms of psychiatric phenomenology. He considered the most significant contributory factors to be stress-related, arguing that:

> '"[I]t was work stress really. I've had manic episodes, or mild ones, all my life at stressful times. I become very paranoid, slightly grandiose, and then [last year], I just had worse episodes." He continued that, in his opinion, "it was work situations that led to it, both, and personal to some extent, so a combination of personal and work situations'.

He clarified that the diagnostic label was given to him by Dr Bryant. He explained he had initially resisted the diagnosis and thought of himself "as having hypomania, which is sort of a below, sub-syndromal condition, so not really, so something you live with without it affecting your life too much, a positive thing if anything". Thus, Alistair did not reject biomedical categories as such, only the particular label attributed to him. His resistance, he continued, was generated by a concern that bipolar disorder "sounded to me like someone with severe mental health issues and, you know, trouble working" and his condition at that point did not seem to be too serious to him. He subsequently experienced his first "severe manic episode" but even then saw this as a "one-off". However, following a second severe episode he changed his view, stating that the bipolar "diagnosis was right".

> 'I think, since I've had the diagnosis of bipolar disorder and had the medication for it, it's become quite straightforward. I think so many people I meet through the mental health services rejected their diagnoses, or feel they've been misdiagnosed. I don't. I read the Wikipedia page on bipolar disorder and think yes, that's exactly what it is like. It feels (a) like a real disease and (b) that that's the right diagnosis. I don't think that many people have that feeling. They feel they just have some symptoms that could be psychiatric or could be

not, so having a diagnosis that fits well like that makes working with Dr Bryant quite easy, because he's seen other people with bipolar and he kind of knows well how, I kind of fit into a category quite well.'

However, returning to his initial disagreement with this diagnosis, Alistair explained that, while he now concurred with it, he had been surprised to discover the label was on his record when he received a copy of a letter from James to his employer. He had believed the question of whether it was hypomania or bipolar disorder had been left open. "I didn't feel like we'd," he paused, then corrected himself, "I'd forgotten that we'd resolved it."

'I remember it coming up and mentioning it to start with, but I don't remember it being, it wasn't discussed like it was a point for discussion. He just assumed that's what it was, and I'd sort of argued against it. It got left and I suppose in my mind I didn't really feel that I'd accepted the diagnosis until six months later or whatever when I had another episode. And then I did.'

But the reaction to the label from some members of Alistair's family worried him. His mother did not accept the notion that he had a mental illness, instead attributing his difficulties to over-tiredness or blaming his wife Felicity for making him "do too many jobs". Alistair explained: "My family haven't really, generally, grasped well that it's a specific disease and that there is not necessarily anyone to blame for anything." In contrast to his mother, Alistair considered factors such as stress to have been a trigger that caused the onset of an acute episode of the underlying disease. The condition, he argued, had a genetic cause. And he identified a grandfather who suffered from depression but may have had a form of bipolar disorder.

Alistair's explanatory framework appears consistent with the stress-vulnerability hypothesis in which environmental factors may trigger an underlying disease entity in genetically predisposed individuals. This contrasts with the familial and environmental explanatory framework that Alistair's mother appeared to have adopted, which, in his view, reinforced blame and stigma. For Alistair, the acceptance of bipolar disorder as a biomedically validated disease entity functioned to reduce this outcome.

Evaluating interventions

Alistair focused in detail on psychological interventions, describing CBT as "useful", reflecting a strong identification with self-help approaches to managing his mental health. However, his view on medication was more ambivalent. Alistair commented that he had been "genuinely happy to try any of the treatments that were available because I was quite in need of help", and this included medication. But he felt, while the olanzapine "really did make a big difference to my mood, it really did bring me down from being, when I was having delusional thoughts, so I think it was very effective. The other medication, I had less proof on that. But [olanzapine] I could feel myself changing after taking it."

Lithium was different. One time, when he was running low on tablets, he made an independent decision to reduce his daily dose from 1000mg to 800mg, as he felt this offered a "natural" opportunity to do so. "I just don't like being on so much medication, just don't like being on long-term medication. I think lithium, you feel is quite a powerful drug to be taking every day, it just doesn't feel right."

However, Alistair later stated that stopping the lithium had been a trigger for one of his "manic episodes", suggesting that he had resigned himself to the rationale for continuing this treatment. Nonetheless, there was a tension between this ambivalence and his later comment about the treatment of bipolar disorder in general: "A psychiatrist friend of a friend said having people with bipolar is quite nice to treat because you can actually make a difference to them, drugs do work, and I think that's true, so it's not just a hopeless case." This faith in the efficacy and utility of biomedical frameworks and treatments, and the hope generated as a result, made it "easy" to work with Dr Bryant "in particular" out of all the other practitioners.

Felicity's perspective

Felicity used a combination of terms to describe Alistair's mental distress. She adopted medical terminology such as the diagnostic label 'bipolar disorder' and utilised the language of 'illness' and 'symptoms', noting that he was "absolutely brilliant at masking" the latter. However, these were interspersed with some dramatically descriptive lay terms. For instance, she described him in the initial stages as "rampaging around ... delusional and, and quite wild really, just manic". He was, she continued: "proper wildly mad, I mean bouncing around the walls, convinced he was being spied on".

Felicity discussed her wish to understand the causal factors underpinning Alistair's mental distress. She explained: "Whenever I ask that question, which I do ask, the psychiatrist will pretty much say that it's random. If I look it up on the internet, people seem to talk about stress being a cause." She clarified that "random" referred to a "chemical imbalance in the brain. But then the care coordinator Filipe will give a different [view]. He thinks Alistair had, is having, a midlife crisis, which isn't a particularly medical view of things. I just hear different things from different people."

She thus identified three main theories of causation that were articulated to account for her husband's experience: a midlife crisis (developmental), stress (environmental) and a chemical imbalance (biological). Felicity strongly rejected the midlife crisis hypothesis, commenting that "it's just one of those things people say, a bit, isn't it, I didn't buy that really". The next theory related to stress. Felicity noted that Alistair had had five "manic episodes" and at least two of these were "very clearly work stress" related. "He had massive, massive things going on at work that would have been enormously stressful to anyone, let alone someone who had a vulnerability to mental health problems." Felicity linked the initial intensification of Alistair's mental health issues to the global financial crisis of 2007–08 and its impact on his work in the insurance industry. But later episodes "seem to have been related to women [at work], some kind of relationship, the beginnings of a relationship or thinking there would be a relationship". Finally, she considered the chemical imbalance hypothesis proposed by James, with a possible related factor being Alistair "messing with his medication", to which she appeared more positively disposed.

However, Felicity explained that it was "hugely frustrating" for her to be exposed to these competing perspectives articulated by different practitioners. For her, resolving these tensions involved "picking the [perspective] that suits your worldview best really. So over time I've learnt whose view most closely matches what my experience is of what is going on". Felicity unequivocally identified James as having the "clearest picture" of Alistair and his needs.

Nonetheless, she later acknowledged the utility of the different perspectives from Filipe and James:

'Because then you can start to think through where you think you sit. Because of course there is no correct answer to what's going on, or what's going to happen next. There's not even a correct answer to the treatment plan, is there? That's the other thing I've learnt about mental health is just how difficult it is to find answers to questions or neat solutions don't exist.'

However, having stated that James's worldview most closely matched her own, and emphasising that this was "in everything really", Felicity paused to reflect on why.

Evaluating interventions

Felicity continued by explaining that Alistair's positive response to medication was the key evidence that underpinned her support for James's perspective. But while Felicity was unequivocal in her support for this approach to treatment, she also advocated a move beyond this individualised approach to consider the wider context of the family system. This was primarily articulated in terms of a sense of frustration with services for failing to satisfactorily engage with her and the children. She explained:

'They weren't interested in having anything to do with the family at all, and that's one of the things I've never understood really about mental health services. How on earth you can treat someone without the context of their family? I find that, and that's still the case now really, and I've battered away at it because I think the impact of the individual's mental health on their immediate family but equally the impact of what's happening to us must also then impact on him again because if we're all in distress it's not going to support him at all and that's happened a lot really to us as a family.'

She thus identified the family as a key systemic context of intervention, noting the potentially significant implications of feedback loops within this setting. Felicity expressed frustration that this "bigger picture" was excluded by the focus on the individual. She was incredulous that "one member of the crisis team suggested I send the kids away while Alistair was ill. That the focus was so much on him that they should be packed and out of the picture is quite extraordinary."

Felicity described James accepting the need to take a more holistic view, but also arguing for deferral of such a family-systems approach during the acute phase. In contrast, Filipe was more oriented to involving Felicity throughout. She explained that during consultations, "Dr Bryant was only really interested in what Alistair said about how he was and not very interested in what I, how I thought Alistair was", while meetings with Filipe were "much more open and very different in nature".

Filipe was:

'just involving me a bit more in the discussion, much less just listening to Alistair, which was what Dr Bryant was doing. He was getting him to talk, for good reasons I think, but it wasn't, he wasn't getting enough of a picture of what was going on by only doing that. You know he's the professional, but I felt he wasn't, and I found it very frustrating really.'

Meanwhile Filipe, she explained, had been "absolutely brilliant at being aware of me as a carer and my perspective on things". While Felicity reasoned that this was a function of the broader role of care coordinator in contrast to the more individual patient-focused doctor, it may also be because of social work's broader social systemic perspective.

Felicity saw herself as engaged in a struggle for recognition of her needs in the work with Alistair. She eventually celebrated the fact that Dr Bryant altered the format of meetings to mirror those with Filipe as a response to this, meeting with Alistair first, before she joined the meeting. "That seemed ideal to me," Felicity stated.

Felicity described a process of learning about services and treatments for Alistair and the family in order to coordinate them more effectively. The aim was to understand "the bigger picture" and achieve better integration of the aspects of treatment. She had done extensive reading, researched on the Royal College of Psychiatry and other websites and talked to a number of people as part of her own wish to better understand mental health problems, treatment options and services following Alistair's diagnosis. But there was a lot of work involved in accessing information about how different services link together and understanding the roles of the various professionals and teams. Moreover, it was difficult to obtain information about the professional affiliation and qualifications of practitioners, unlike counsellors in private practice where extensive information was readily available online.

Felicity was also frustrated that she needed to identify and self-refer to services for her and the children, for instance family therapy for her daughter and the 'Kids Time' support and information group for all her children. This reflected one of the key issues Felicity identified: the tendency to devolve decision making and responsibility to the carer. Over time, as she developed an understanding, she felt compelled to respond more assertively:

'Alistair was discharged wrongly in many ways. He was sectioned and then discharged after six days. He was still incredibly ill but none of us realised. Well, I tried to hand Alistair over to mental health services because he was lapdancing at night and all these things and he wasn't living at home. And I was just, like, you lot deal with him.'

She laughed. "Until it turned out that it wasn't being done very well and then I felt I had to come back in and make sure things were being done properly." The extent of Felicity's developing expertise around medical interventions became apparent when she resolved inconsistencies in relation to medication advice. She described a discussion around the use of the antipsychotic, olanzapine, where Alistair was getting mixed messages from the Crisis Resolution Team. She "had to prod again because the Crisis Team were saying: 'Oh well, if you don't want to take it don't.' But Dr Bryant had said very clearly he should take it. So I had to prod them again to say: 'You've got to take this [olanzapine].' And it worked."

This reflects Felicity's adoption of a citizen-consumer role (Clarke et al, 2007; Rogers et al, 2009). She skilfully accessed information, for instance via books and websites, while articulating the need for more consumer-related data to support choices for Alistair, herself and their children. She navigated competing conceptions of mental distress within this interdisciplinary environment and drew on her experiential knowledge to arrive at judgements regarding treatment options.

While a greater role for carers is often described in terms of empowerment, this trend reflects the devolving of responsibility from the state to individuals and their families in the context of neoliberal welfare retrenchment (Clarke et al, 2007). It is then that the personal resources on which the citizen-consumer is able to draw, which are socially and structurally positioned, become more significant. Felicity knew that the family were "middle class and articulate". At first she saw this as a barrier to accessing statutory services following treatment in the private sector funded by Alistair's employer. But eventually they were "swamped" with services, including unusually frequent contact with the consultant psychiatrist, care coordinator and senior psychologist.[7] Felicity also mentioned being able to draw on advice from her immediate network, which included her brother-in-law, a surgeon and a friend who is a psychologist. This suggested access to social capital commensurate with her class background.

As Felicity developed her knowledge, she felt able to more actively engage with decision-making contexts and processes. An example was a four-page letter she wrote to James to articulate her concerns regarding Alistair's treatment. She regarded this as a positive turning point in her relationship with this practitioner and with services. She felt a growing sense of agency because, as she noted, services and practitioners "will adapt themselves to what you want".

Filipe's perspective

In the interviews, social worker Filipe began by emphasising his rejection of a biomedical framework for Alistair:

'Even though I appreciate, you know, psychiatry and the medical model, I wouldn't really necessarily use that kind of intervention really, because I think, at the end of the day, [with Alistair] there's no sort of history, there's not [a] kind of a genetic sort of predisposition there. I really truly believe that is pretty much kind of an impact of the environment and also the kind of lifestyle that he led.'

Filipe drew attention to alternative social and environmental factors:

'I have learnt so much about his mental health issues not only in terms of the complexity of relationship within family, immediate family not necessarily, not talking about his wife and his kids but also his stepfather and mother, and also there are the two brothers and a sister. I learnt quite a lot about the expectations that people have on him in terms of status, financial situation and the demands that people have imposed onto him since he was a teenager. And there is no history in the family of *any* sort of mental health issues from both parts, from his mum's side or his father's side.'

In foregrounding these two related social factors – complex family relationships and the pressure of status expectations from Alistair's middle-class background – Filipe was keen to emphasise the absence of a family history of mental illness. This functioned to undermine the claims for the significance of genetic heredity utilised by advocates of biomedical frameworks. This formed a significant contrast with the identification by James earlier of a first-degree relative (mother or brother) with schizophrenia. This matter is of considerable import within the domain of psychiatry where a family history of schizophrenia is regarded as the primary risk factor for this condition (Gottesman, 1991). Alistair's own position did not assist in adjudicating between these accounts because, although he aligned with the genetic position, he identified only a second-degree relative (grandfather) and was not confident of the diagnosis attributed to him. These divergences illuminate the way in which competing professional interests construct diverse objects of scrutiny in this contested field.

Filipe thought the pressure of Alistair's high-status job was "detrimental to his mental health". His preoccupation with work, and related levels of stress, had particularly damaging consequences for relationships with his family, in particular his wife. One work-related concern arising during recent episodes involved sexual advances made by Alistair to female colleagues at work. Filipe thought this was a midlife crisis. "There is a mix of also, you know, kind of a middle-aged guy, questioning about what he's done in his life, who he is, what he is up to, what he's done or not done and I want to be young again." Thus, Filipe drew on a range of social, environmental and developmental factors to explain the aetiology of Alistair's mental health issues, with a particular focus on the role of family, status and employment stressors.

Filipe defined his own framework in opposition to that of the medical diagnostic model offered by James. He argued: "We need to work as well by individual cases. We have to be careful not just to generalise for the sake of, you know, that's what the book says." For Filipe, diagnosis represented the reduction of the range and diversity of human experience to the categories defined in key biomedical psychiatric texts such as the *Diagnostic and Statistical Manual of Mental Disorders* (American Psychiatric Association, 2013).

The differences between Filipe and James had the potential to develop into open conflict within multiprofessional meetings. Filipe explained:

'I agree to disagree with his consultant, you know, and I think vice versa. I did mention sort of once at CPA [Care Programme Approach] meetings or kind of a meeting that I had with Alistair, his wife and the consultant, that I, you know, I do really believe that, you know, so it's kind of a baggage, it's also a mid–life crisis that he is going through. The consultant, of course, is pretty much kind of: "No, this is bipolar disorder, that's what happens." And I said: "Of course it is, but we can't label it as regards that." He has acquired that at the age of 40 something, it's kind of late in the stage of his life, compared to many others, as much as I remember about research that I've read about it.'

Filipe's critique of James's categorisation of Alistair's mental health needs as bipolar disorder had two strands. The first hinted at the problematic elements of labelling. The second rejected James's perspective from within its own medical terms of reference by appealing to research evidence that invalidated this diagnosis as a result of the late onset of Alistair's condition.

Filipe said that he "wouldn't use the diagnostic label bipolar disorder myself, I think especially being trained and professionally, I wouldn't really". He thus invoked professional authority as support for the rejection of this category. I asked if he would use any particular alternative term.

'I'm not sure really. It's a really interesting discussion, because I do have to acknowledge that, yes, there's an element of that. But I don't think that this is it for him, even though once you're labelled with something like that, it's quite difficult to detach from it, you know. And severe enduring mental illness for the rest of your life, I mean, is part of it. I'm not sure really, you know, hypomanic, there's so many different terminologies really and I suppose really, for myself, maybe I'm kidding myself, but I'd like to say that he is going through still a very difficult midlife crisis too. But it's not just that. I acknowledge maybe the rest of it. It's a difficult question to answer to be honest.'

Here Filipe modulated his position, acknowledging that there was an 'element' of validity in the diagnosis. But he restated his concerns around labelling and identified the stigma arising from this. He tentatively proposed the alternative term 'hypomanic' to describe Alistair's experiences. The latter term, while still positioned within a medical discourse, evokes a liminal state between 'normality' and 'mental illness' that is somewhat less subject to psychiatric intervention and is, therefore, a space where psychosocial responses carry greater legitimacy.

This section started with a focus on contrasts between Filipe and James in the way they understood Alistair's needs. But while tensions and conflicts accompany interprofessional teamworking between psychiatrists and social workers, and other professional groups in teams, there are also complex ambivalences. Here we saw shifts in Filipe's position between outright rejection, uncertainty and equivocation in relation to both the diagnosis of bipolar disorder and the broader medical diagnostic process.

Strategies for intervention 1: talking therapy and practical support

Filipe used two main strands of intervention with Alistair: "practical work" and "talking therapy". Filipe explained that he was not a qualified marriage counsellor, but he had "substantial experience" in this field. So his interventions included work to address the difficulties, anger and resentment around Alistair's absence from the family due to heavy work commitments, his dependence on his wife's social networks, his conduct with colleagues at work and his management of stress. Filipe explained that he particularly enjoyed this work for the opportunity to look beyond the individual casework model.

Filipe used a number of models of psychological intervention, including humanistic approaches such as "Carl Rogers, but also problem solving" and CBT. For instance, on the day of the interview, Filipe had met with Alistair and described using the type of scaling questions utilised in CBT to elicit his mood. But Filipe was eager to explain that he was not duplicating interventions by the psychologist, Spencer. "I want to work on, not only sort of on the feelings, the sentiments, if you like, about fear, anxiety, recognition of, you know, his own ability to do things or not, self-esteem, but also the practicalities."

Filipe reluctantly conceded that "medication has helped". But he was also concerned that Alistair was:

'having 1000mg lithium, he has citalopram, he has aripiprazole and I think something else. It's a cocktail. So there's a mood stabiliser, the other is antidepressant, so it's like a yo-yo inside his brains, you know, really messing about so much, you know that you can't try to stabilise, so it's like, I think, he's never said this, but he's feeling, I think, like a kind of a guinea pig.'

Thus, for Filipe, the iatrogenic potentials of the medication regime were problematic and psychological intervention formed the key emphasis in his work. "In terms of intervention really, I believe that actually the best one here is talking therapy."

Strategies for intervention 2: managing 'higher risk' periods

Initially Filipe went to great lengths to differentiate his approach from that of James, drawing a strong contrast between James's biological and his own social and environmental perspective on aetiology, and between the 'cocktail' of medication prescribed by James and his own advocacy of talking therapies. However, this differentiation was challenged when Alistair entered a period Filipe called a time of "higher risk", and James called the 'acute phase'.

This contrast became apparent when, later in the interview, I enquired whether issues of risk played a role in shaping Filipe's understanding of mental health needs and choice of interventions. I made brief reference to a serious violent incident a few days before, involving another CMHT service user, Patrick, who was apparently the perpetrator. Filipe was Patrick's care coordinator, and I asked him whether he also drew on humanistic Rogerian and cognitive approaches in his work with this service user.

'Yes, I did use very, pretty much similar approaches, in terms of the kind of, you know, kind of a role of a counsellor too, and sort of listening, reflecting and I'm using sort of lots of, kind of a warmth approach and stuff like this. However, this particular other case [Patrick] really, it's always been, the risk factors are extremely high. Because there's been a huge history, sort of psychiatric history in the family. And this this guy, lots of violence really. So with him, I was always fully aware about his needs … But I'm not sure … I'm thinking because he was staying in supported accommodation, at Avenue House, the local one here, that I didn't really spend as much time, because I thought he was in a much, kind of a safe environment, that he had the support there.

And this guy [Alistair] was on his own even though he had lots of support from the wife. But in terms of risk factors really, kind of when I say suicidal ideation or anything like that, well, we need to be careful. Because the indication was really, the risk factors were getting pretty much higher and higher and higher and higher. So, you know, he became really psychotic and very delusional, very paranoid. And I'm not quite sure if he's got dual diagnosis really, schizophrenia and bipolar, because … one day he could only see sort of elderly people in the street or only gay people … so very delusional, very kind of, very troubled, very unwell. I do tend to really worry about, more … about people [with] a dual diagnosis.'

Here Filipe's register shifted dramatically as issues of risk came into focus. He described how his assessment of risk was guided by factors that included Patrick's family psychiatric history, which typically implied genetic inheritance. He then described the necessity to choose among competing priorities. He described his judgement that risk (to others) was adequately managed in Patrick's case because of placement in staffed, supported accommodation. This was in contrast to Alistair's risk (to himself), which was escalating dramatically and more difficult to manage because Alistair had separated from his wife and was living alone in temporary accommodation.

For Filipe, a key element in the evaluation and attribution of higher levels of risk was whether someone has a 'dual diagnosis'. Alistair was described as a candidate for inclusion in this category as he had reported considering every person he encountered to be gay or elderly. Filipe had considered this implausible in those contexts and therefore adjudged these to constitute "paranoid" and "delusional" ideas, possibly indicating "schizophrenia", and thus, in Filipe's words, a "dual diagnosis" in combination with "bipolar".

This extract stands in stark contrast to Filipe's position on diagnosis elaborated earlier. Here he mobilised psychiatric terminology and diagnostic categories extensively to describe the mental health of both Alistair and Patrick, only intermittently using a non-medicalised vocabulary such as 'troubled' to describe Alistair's mental health. The legitimation of medicalised strategies was also apparent in the type of intervention recommended by Filipe during this 'higher risk' stage:

'As you know, men at that age to be diagnosed with bipolar, the risk factors are very high really in terms of suicide and risk to themselves and to others. So we had crisis team involved, crisis house. We had psychology involved, therapists, we had myself looking into [a] therapeutic relationship with the guy and also my role as a social worker. And I think six months later he improved a lot, he stabilised his mood, complied with medication, seeing the consultant here on a very regular basis.'

There appeared to be a marked shift in emphasis by Filipe during this 'higher risk' or 'acute' stage, and much greater convergence between Filipe and James in terms of analysis of the most appropriate forms of intervention.

Work-related stress, social class and situational logics

This chapter highlights two important themes. The first is the way that dominant situational logics generate directional tendencies in practice that relegate considerations of social-structural processes to the margins within mental health services. As Felicity noted, the global financial crash caused "massive, massive" stress for Alistair in his role as a senior executive in finance. However, this major social stressor, although acknowledged by all, was relatively peripheral to James and Filipe's reflections on the causes of Alistair's mental distress. This is despite employment being one of the central contexts of adult social experience, and growing recognition of the links between mental distress and the effects of wider socioeconomic structures, such as the organisation of work and (conflictual) social relations within workplaces (Fenwick and Tausig, 2007).[8] The reason for this is that, as with factors relating to racialised inequalities explored in the previous chapter, dominant situational logics under neoliberalism have created strategic directional tendencies that marginalise such structural considerations. Instead, the prioritisation of issues of *risk* within a particular institutional hierarchy (*medical dominance*) tends to foreground *custodial* and *biomedical* interventions.

The second key theme is the significance of service users' experiences of transitions between 'stable' and 'acute' phases of mental distress in making more visible the operation of these changing situational logics and directional tendencies. As this chapter has illustrated, Filipe was critical of James's biomedical stance during Alistair's stable phases, focusing on providing therapeutic and more systemic family-oriented support (*social-relational approaches*). However, he shifted noticeably when this service user's levels of distress and suicide *risk* increased (the acute phase). At this stage, Filipe appropriated a more diagnostic vocabulary and aligned more closely with James's proposal (*medical dominance*) for *biomedical model* treatments within the inpatient setting (*custodialism*). This illustrates the effects of a changing situational logic that emerged as Alistair moved into a 'crisis' phase, which was generated by a combination of the four emergent features noted above (*risk, medical dominance, custodial* and *biomedical interventions*). This created a directional tendency towards custodial paternalism, which manifested through Filipe's realignment of his conceptual and practical stance on Alistair's needs in response to these directional pressures.

Punitive managerialism under austerity

The previous four chapters described the effects of the neoliberal restructuring of Southville Community Mental Health Team (CMHT) during the first phase of data collection. Between then and the second phase, there were three key areas of policy reform and service transformation. These were: austerity-related funding constraints within local authorities and the National Health Service (NHS); welfare reform; and the service-line management (SLM) reorganisation of team structures and service delivery within the Trust. This chapter, based on the second phase of data collection, will examine these processes and their effects, in particular how service provision became more short term and the managerial culture more punitive following the transition to a Rehabilitation and Recovery Team (RRT) structure.

The policy context of service transformation

The austerity agenda and funding constraints

In Chapter 1, three phases of neoliberal mental health policy and service delivery reforms were identified, with the most recent – the austerity phase – beginning to emerge from 2009. However, this policy agenda was dramatically escalated and deepened with the election of the Conservative–Liberal coalition government in 2010. Impacts on the health and social care sectors were significant. The NHS was faced with a combination of unprecedented funding constraints amid rising demand. This led to a substantial funding gap, while the social care sector experienced even greater relative spending reductions (Stoye, 2017; Watkins et al, 2017).

In NHS statutory mental health services, during 2011/12, the coalition government presided over a cut in funding for the first time in a decade. Most mental health providers continued to face falling income throughout its term (Gilburt, 2016). NHS Mental Health Trusts sought to manage this funding crisis through strategies such as reductions in levels of staffing and inpatient provision (Gilburt, 2015).[1] At the national level there was a 13 per cent fall in the number of full-time-equivalent mental health nurses between 2009 and 2017 – that includes a reduction in the number of more experienced nurses (Gilburt, 2018) – and a 30 per cent cut in the number of inpatient beds between 2009 and 2018 (Helm and Campbell, 2018). At the local level, within the NHS Trust under study here there was an 18 per cent cut in the number of nurses between 2011 and 2014,[2] one of the highest figures in the country, and a reduction in total inpatient beds from 365 to 235 between 2007 and 2017, a fall of 35 per cent.[3] This led to an escalation of practices such as 'out-of-area' placements (OAPs), which have been shown to have detrimental impacts for the experience of service users (Trewin, 2017). Locally, during the 2011–14 period, the number of service users subject to OAPs rose from 89 to 171.[4]

In addition to the NHS funding squeeze, there has been an even more dramatic fall in local authority budgets. Central government imposed unprecedented cumulative cuts of almost half (49.1 per cent) in grants to local authorities between 2010/11 and 2017/18, resulting in a £7 billion drop in local authority spending on adult social care during this period (National Audit Office, 2018; ADASS, 2019). This has had a significant impact on mental health provision because NHS Trusts in mental health are funded and delivered via partnership arrangements between the NHS and local government. Community services such as day centres, reablement and other forms of adult social care support are also funded by local authorities.

The detrimental impact of austerity measures on NHS and local authority mental health service provision became increasingly visible during the latter stages of the coalition government. Public concerns about cuts led to greater scrutiny, and in some places, campaigns, frequently led by service users but also involving practitioners and other allies, to challenge service closures and funding constraints (Moth et al, 2015).

In this context of higher levels of public concern about and criticism of the state of mental health services, the government set up an independent Mental Health Taskforce (2016), which went on to produce a set of policy proposals: *The Five Year Forward View for Mental Health*. Following this, mechanisms that purport to monitor and address underfunding and associated challenges in mental health services have been introduced. But problems associated with slow funding growth and insufficient staffing levels remain (Gilburt, 2018). These have placed enormous strains on mental health workers and have had significant implications for the nature, quality and accessibility of support offered to service users.

Welfare reform

A central focus of neoliberal reform of the welfare state during the austerity era has been the benefits system. The reform programme here has two main components. One is reductions in levels of social security support and increased conditionality (Patrick, 2017). Examples include the 2010 coalition government's below-inflation uprating of benefits, followed by a benefit rate freeze under the 2015 Conservative administration (Beatty and Fothergill, 2016). The other is restriction of access to welfare benefits by redrawing eligibility boundaries (Roulstone, 2015).

Reforms to two welfare benefit measures were particularly relevant for mental health service users. One is Employment and Support Allowance

(ESA), an out-of-work benefit introduced in 2008 for people experiencing illness or incapacity. This is assessed via the controversial work capability assessment, and is the main income replacement benefit for disabled claimants or those with ill-health. The other is Personal Independence Payment (PIP), a non-means-tested extra-costs benefit for people with a long-term physical or mental health condition or impairment, introduced from 2013 to replace Disability Living Allowance for claimants aged 16–64. Universal Credit had also just been introduced locally at the time of data collection.

Another significant trend in reform has been a 'welfare-to-work' orientation facilitated by escalating conditionality. This emerged in the early 2000s during the New Labour era and further intensified under the Conservative-led coalition government. For instance, conditions were extended to in-work benefit recipients; a situation characterised as 'ubiquitous conditionality'. A prominent form of welfare conditionality involves 'behavioural conduct' conditions, such as requirements to engage in job searching, mandatory courses or workfare (Dwyer and Wright, 2014).

However, 'psychological conditionality' has also become an increasingly integral feature of welfare-to-work regimes (Watts and Fitzpatrick, 2018). This goes beyond conduct requirements by demanding claimants modify their attitudes, dispositions or personality in order to return to or find work. This is underpinned by the notion of unemployment as a product of individual psychological deficits (Friedli and Stearn, 2015). The escalation of various types of conditionality has been combined with sanctions for non-compliance, representing an increasingly 'punitive turn' in UK welfare provision (Taylor-Gooby, 2016; Fletcher and Wright, 2018).

Also visible is a much greater alignment of mental health policy with the welfare-to-work agenda that is an integral feature of 'supply-side' neoliberal social policy (Moth and McKeown, 2016; McKenna et al, 2019). This is apparent in the notion of 'employment as a health outcome' foregrounded in the *Five Year Forward View* policy document. This has manifested as a government-imposed performance indicator requiring NHS Trusts to double the number of service users accessing employment-related support (Mental Health Taskforce, 2016). Measures to address the iniquities of the disability employment gap are welcome. But some mental health service user activists regard this agenda as a 'work cure' extension of punitive workfare, rather than an attempt to address structural barriers and discrimination in the labour market (Frayne, 2019; McKenna et al, 2019).

Service-line management: from CMHT to Rehabilitation and Recovery Team

Service reconfigurations have become an important way for NHS Trusts to manage reduced income during the austerity era (Gilburt, 2015). From

2012, in the mental health context, this took the form of service-line management (SLM).

At this time, as Chapter 1 noted, the Mental Health Payments System (MHPS) was introduced to replace block contracts for service provision with an approach based on individual care pathways. These pathways represent costed 'business units' of provision that facilitate a process of deepening commodification of mental health services. This care pathway approach has been implemented through SLM organisational restructuring of NHS Mental Health Trusts. The new SLM care pathways are oriented around the 21 clusters of 'need' identified in the Health of the Nation Outcome Scale (HoNOS) (DH Payment by Results Team, 2012). The assessment of a service user using HoNOS tools enables identification of the appropriate cluster of need associated with a particular care pathway (service line) to which the user is then allocated (Twomey et al, 2015). Each of the 21 clusters is grouped within one of the three broad 'super-classes' of care pathway: non-psychotic, psychosis and organic. While these 'needs' clusters are not based on specific psychiatric diagnoses, it is argued that combining diagnostic data with care pathways improves the reliability of clusters for costing purposes (Kingdon et al, 2012).

Moreover, in practice guidance, certain diagnostic categories are explicitly associated with particular clusters. For instance, clusters within the *non-psychotic* super-class indicate likely primary diagnoses such as anxiety disorder and depressive episode, *psychosis* clusters suggest possible primary diagnoses like schizophrenia and bipolar disorder, while primary diagnoses such as dementia are frequently seen in the *organic* super-cluster (NHS Improvement, 2019).

New multidisciplinary team formats with a more specialised focus were created and introduced across England from 2012 onwards, in order to align with this suite of policy reforms (Kalidindi et al, 2012). The SLM model eschews the more generic approach symbolised by the old CMHT, where service users with a diverse range of mental health needs were supported within the same service. The new system groups together services for people with putative similarities in type of mental health need. At Southville, SLM restructuring led not only to the merger of Southville CMHT with two other teams, but its reconfiguration into a new Rehabilitation and Recovery Team (RRT) located within the psychosis service line. This meant that service users with primary diagnostic labels such as personality disorder were transferred across to teams within other service lines or discharged. The new RRT focused solely on those with so-called psychotic disorders. RRTs primarily support service users whose needs are assessed as 'ongoing or recurrent psychosis' with low symptoms (cluster 11), with high disability (cluster 12) or with high symptoms and disability (cluster 13) (Jacobs, 2014).

Alongside increased specialisation in relation to user needs, there has also been a contraction in the range of core tasks. For instance, previously each CMHT had its own structure for assessing new referrals. But since the reorganisation this function has been centralised within a new service-wide Assessment and Advice Team, now based in primary care. This new team conducts initial assessments and manages referrals into all Trust services, including the RRT.

Experiences of neoliberal service transformations

Southville: from CMHT to RRT

The new RRT that emerged as a result of these SLM reforms replaced three CMHTs, including Southville. The structure of the new RRT was as follows: one team manager (from a community mental health nurse – CMHN – background), two deputy managers (one social worker and one occupational therapist), six CMHNs, five social workers, three clinical psychologists (2.5 full-time-equivalent [FTE] posts) and five support workers. The team was supported by two part-time workers, one focused on welfare rights (0.6 FTE) and the other on employment support (0.5 FTE). The team worked with one consultant psychiatrist, one ST5 (SpR) and one ST3 (SHO senior house officer). As this suggests, the RRT was broadly similar in size to Southville CMHT in terms of core team numbers. The most visible changes were an increase in team capacity in relation to clinical psychology, the addition of support workers and employment support workers, and a cut in welfare rights capacity.

Although this appears to be a modest increase in RRT staffing levels when compared with one community mental health team, these changes in fact represented a significant decrease overall when compared with the three teams that were replaced. In terms of service user numbers, the admission criteria for the RRT are narrower than those for the CMHT, with RRT eligibility limited to users allocated to clusters 11–13 (that is, the 'psychosis' service lines for those with diagnoses such as schizophrenia, bipolar disorder and so on). Trust documents identify that, at the point of the restructure, 66 per cent of CMHT service users met the diagnostic eligibility criteria for RRT.[5] Broadly speaking, then, the RRT has just over a third of the staffing levels of the three CMHTs it replaced but with a remit to cover two thirds of the user population formerly served by them.

Of the Southville CMHT practitioner participants from the first phase of the study, only community mental health nurse (CMHN) Kath, social workers Yvonne, Ruth and Farooq, and welfare rights worker Martin continued to work in the RRT. Team manager Evelyn and nurse Roger both retired. Other team members, including nurse Leslie,[6] left the Trust for posts in alternative welfare service settings. All of the practitioners listed here, except Farooq, participated in the second phase of data collection.[7] However, unfortunately, due to time and resource constraints, it was not possible to negotiate access to offer first-phase service user participants the opportunity to participate in the second phase of the study. This is an extremely significant omission with considerable implications for the findings. However, data collection and analysis during this phase have been informed by other recent studies I have conducted involving mental health service user participants reflecting on their lived experiences of service use and welfare provision (Moth et al, 2015; Moth and Lavalette, 2017; Moth et al, 2018). By doing so, I have sought to ensure, as far as possible, that the issues articulated by service user participants in those studies inform the analysis and arguments developed here.

The next section will explore practitioners' perspectives on the SLM reconfiguration, associated changes in the labour process and the implications for workers and service users. Service-line restructuring of the labour process has accelerated and deepened the relational to informational trends that were already visible within the old CMHT. Moreover, participants described an increasingly punitive, command-and-control oriented managerial culture in the Trust, with experiences of stress and bullying common for staff, and increasingly limited and short-term interventions for users.

Reconfiguring the RRT labour process and service provision

Participants identified four pertinent dimensions of the reconfigured labour process. At the organisational level, there was the restructuring of the RRT workforce and the recomposition of the service user population. At the interpersonal (micro) level there was a reorientation of practice modalities and changing temporalities of practice.

Restructuring the RRT workforce

Chapter 2 highlighted two key dimensions of the reorganisation of the division of labour within the CMHT workforce: deskilling/specialisation and labour substitution. The reconfiguration further embedded these trends. A third dimension was the deletion or *downbanding* of frontline posts held by more experienced practitioners (in particular from nursing, numerically the largest occupational group within the Trust). Downbanding involves the pay band for a role being reduced by the employer (Jones-Berry, 2016).

Leslie described how all the nursing and occupational therapist practitioners in Southville CMHT had "to reapply for our posts, which were all downgraded to band six posts". This process involved interviews, then a written assessment. All those frontline workers at Southville who had applied managed to secure RRT posts (CMHT manager Evelyn was the exception to this – her experiences will be presented in the next chapter). But, Leslie said: "I know in other teams there were people that didn't get posts." And the process created an unwelcome sense of "competition among us all". CMHN Kath, relatively close to retirement, said the downbanding left her feeling "resentful", not only due to lower pay but also "because … I've lost out on my pension". She had already experienced a gendered penalty for working part-time during much of her career due to childcare commitments, and downbanding further compounded this loss.

Many participants described feeling that experienced professionals were no longer considered to be a vital resource by NHS Trusts. For instance, during the first phase of fieldwork, as the SLM changes approached, Crisis Team CMHN Simon had expressed concern that the purpose of the Trust's deletion of senior nursing posts was to save money in the context of austerity. However, this had significant implications for service delivery, he explained, because long-serving practitioners such as Leslie had built up significant "street knowledge" of both local services and the needs of service users over many years of practice. This was an important resource that benefitted service users, Simon argued, but which no longer seemed to be valued by Trust senior managers.

The other trajectories, towards deskilling, specialisation and labour substitution, were also further extended through SLM. Labour substitution was visible in the recruitment of a new tier of lower-paid (Band 4) support workers to the RRT.[8] This skill-mix reform enabled the redistribution of practitioners' workloads to reduce costs, the internal equivalent of external outsourcing. For Kath, issues of control as well as cost underpinned the Trust's motivation for recruiting this new tier of support workers. They were "not only cheaper, they're younger and tend not to be so gobby [outspoken]. They're less confident [and can be] herded and chewed up."

Practitioners also described a more punitive atmosphere at work, driven by an increasingly draconian managerial culture within the Trust. Welfare rights worker Martin said: "The management style is much more top heavy, much more authoritarian, much more dictatorial than it used to be. I mean, it's like we're not in this together, you do what I tell you." Following the SLM reorganisation, CMHT manager Evelyn was moved out of her post. CMHN Leslie described the first RRT manager after Evelyn as "a whipcracker, big time, you know, around about things like punctuality and sickness and so on, which just caused further anxiety within the team".

For social worker Steve, these trends were actively inculcated within training courses for NHS managers, who were encouraged "to be distant from the workers, not to be too friendly and to just basically carry on as if they're in a business environment". Martin concurred. He said there had been a shift in "the ideological stance of the people who are actually managing the services. They're buying into these kinds of agendas. So, it's partly about the funding and the money, it's also partly about the philosophy, the thinking behind it. There's been a dramatic shift to an agenda of market principles."

One example is a conversation among team members about the Trust's former medical director, the most senior psychiatrist in the organisation,

Ruth (social worker):	'He was the one that made the decision to cut the beds.'
Kath (nurse):	'And then went into private healthcare.'
Ruth:	'Yeah, so he cut all those beds, which forced the Trust to pay for private beds and then, lo and behold, he goes and gets a top job at a private company.'
Steve (social worker):	'It's shocking really.'
Leslie (nurse):	'At [Psy-Beds Ltd],[9] where some of those [NHS] beds would be outsourced to.'

This highlights the 'revolving door' for senior managers between the public and private healthcare sectors, with very significant attendant conflicts of financial interest. Practitioners also felt that the market philosophy was filtering further down within the organisation. Kath noted that "the managers with these philosophies used to be the top-level managers running the Trust. Now it's our team managers that have this business ethos and have that disconnect" from workers and users. As a result of this disconnect, team managers "don't know what we're doing on a day-to-day basis or the stresses around it, they don't know what we do and how we do it and how that affects us, no idea".

For Leslie, the new style of management contrasted with an older form that sought to "protect the team from the worst excesses of the targets and stats-driven culture". Evelyn thought these protective "old school" managers had been "professional leaders who kind of had those values of professionalism at their heart and then took on the management role". This more collegiate managerial approach,[10] which involved supporting practitioners' professional development, including relational and therapeutic aspects of practice, had given way to a greater emphasis on enforcing the Trust's informational demands. To fulfil this latter requirement, Kath argued, "the managers now are very much 'yes men' in hitting the targets".

Social worker Yvonne noted that spaces such as supervision meetings between team members and their line manager had previously offered opportunities for reflection and professional development but were now "led by bringing your [targets] dashboard out and what needs to be done". As a result, Kath argued, practitioners' experiences of managerial control in the Trust were characterised by "stresses and bullying conditions".

Overall, the CMHT to RRT reconfiguration was a painful transition for both the Trust workforce and this particular team. It involved both significant reductions in workers' terms and conditions to deliver cost savings and a shift to more draconian modes of managerial control. Although the SLM reorganisation represented an extension and deepening of trends that were already visible in the latter years of the CMHT, practitioners regarded the RRT changes as a tipping point in market-oriented reform.

RRT and recomposition of the service user population

The SLM reconfiguration had significant implications for service users as well as mental health workers. SLM led to more restricted eligibility criteria for the RRT than the CMHT. This 'fragmentation through specialisation' reflects wider neoliberalising trends in the welfare state (Baldwin, 2009; Carey, 2015; Featherstone et al, 2018). In this context, the focus on clusters 11–13, known as the 'psychosis' service line, narrowed the scope of the team and meant a reduced 'caseload mix' for practitioners. This heralded two major and interrelated changes in service provision for many service users: discharge and duty.

CMHN Leslie described how, in the early stages of the transition from CMHT to RRT, "there was a lot of pressure to discharge people, despite them having perhaps significant vulnerabilities". This 'throughput' approach contrasted with the CMHT where "we would probably have worked with them ongoing". The rationale for the raising of thresholds for access in this way appeared to be linked to the sheer volume of demand in the context of reduced service provision arising from the CMHT to RRT transition. As Leslie explained, "there was a real sense of the Trust moving clients towards discharge so that we could prioritise other clients who were coming into the service".

A clinical zoning (traffic-light) system was utilised at the RRT to facilitate these discharge-focused processes. Leslie explained that "quite a lot of clients were discharged or were moved on to what was called 'red team', which was a part of the intake system, and they were then followed up through a sort of duty-type system for a period of time". This duty system therefore functioned as a 'step down' from care coordination for many service users, a reduction to 'crisis-only' support from the RRT that was intended to be a staging point towards discharge.

However, for Leslie, this widespread discharging strategy entailed significant risks for a section of the service user population. To illustrate this, he described one service user who had a "history of sort of depression with psychotic features, had significant physical health problems, wasn't able to both recognise and manage them, and was very frightened of hospitals and medical procedures. There was always a bit of a pressure to discharge him." Leslie had nonetheless advocated for ongoing support for the service user and assessments by psychiatrists had tended to concur with this view until 2014 when Leslie left the team. At this point, the service user was discharged along with four other users from Leslie's caseload with similarly complex needs.

> 'I know that within a year or two, some of those clients passed away. I wouldn't say in any way that they passed away as a consequence of the system. I can't make that call really. But you just think if, when their physical health did deteriorate, if someone was continuing to go in periodically and pick up the idiosyncrasies of their personality and their mental health problem. Might that person have got another spell of treatment in hospital and sustained life for a longer period of time?'

Leslie was careful not to claim a direct causal link between discharge and these service users' deaths. However, other practitioners shared his concern about a potential link between these tragic outcomes and the prevailing institutional tendency towards 'psychiatric neglect' (Spandler, 2016) in the context of austerity.[11]

Evelyn recounted a similar scenario described to her by Ruth, who had recently visited a service user as part of her duty role. This service user was 'held' on the duty system and therefore only "halfish attached to services", and when Ruth arrived, she found he had "died of physical health problems, alone, in a flat". Like Leslie, Evelyn did not assert a direct link between this death and reduced support under duty but did suggest that such outcomes became more likely in a context of greater organisational neglect. She argued that during the CMHT era, service users such as those described by Ruth and Leslie might have been offered alternatives to this 'discharge or duty' approach.

Evelyn described what she termed "backburner" clients, evoking the analogy of "the pot at the back of the stove". She explained that, formerly, discussions among CMHT team members might identify service users who, although not currently in crisis, expressed or invited some level of concern among practitioners or from the service user themselves about their readiness for discharge. In so far as the team could identify "good, coherent, clinical reasons for not discharging", they would offer ongoing although less frequent levels of contact, thus reducing the likelihood of 'psychiatric neglect'.

The implementation of SLM has led to a significant recomposition of the service user population served by the RRT, due to the new HoNOS cluster-based eligibility criteria. However, this recomposition is also a product of the reorientation in the RRT towards 'throughput' and stepped care, which is institutionalised in the emphasis on discharge and expanded role for the duty system. As we have seen, many practitioners regarded these changes as leading to increased levels of institutional neglect in the system.

Reorienting modalities of practice

A prominent change in the labour process of mental health workers arising from the SLM restructure was that a significantly increased proportion of the face-to-face work of the team was now carried out in the context of 'duty work' rather than through long-term care coordination. Duty is a system for supporting and managing service users who have been accepted by the RRT but are not yet care coordinated due to a shortage of capacity among practitioners. Duty also serves a smaller number of previously care-coordinated service users who have been 'stepped down' to this status as part of a transition towards discharge from the team. RRT members are rostered to provide duty cover at certain points during their working hours, typically around one day per week.

Relational work: from depth to surface

Social worker Yvonne described the merger of CMHTs during the restructure: "Although we lost a lot of staff, the same amount of clients remained, meaning that duty became a holding ground for clients who were unallocated and that's still the case today. We have a large number of clients and those clients have been held on duty." Related to this was the reduction by the Trust of the average RRT care coordination caseload from 25 (the typical CMHT figure) to 20 service users per full-time worker. However, CMHN Kath explained that "that's a caseload reduction, it's not work reduction", because the work of RRT practitioners was being reoriented towards supporting service users within the duty system.

As a result, welfare rights worker Martin argued that the nature of work had "definitely changed". There was a higher turnover of service users. "A lot more stuff is dealt with via duty. It's much more crisis management than it used to be. The old school care coordination, keeping in close touch, people just don't have the time to do that anymore." Similarly, social worker Yvonne noted that care coordination-type tasks were now being carried out on duty. "The work is very different now. The continuity of care and work, it can't be managed really. Duty becomes so busy because you might be seeing four or five clients who you don't know."

Nurse Kath described the high volume of work on a typical duty shift:

'There would probably be a ward round, a home visit or somebody coming in, phone calls and it can get quite, quite busy. New clients, home visits, sometimes it would be about getting face-to-face assessments or PIP [Personal Independence Payment] assessments, chasing up housing, social care packages, that kind of thing. Its very task orientated.'

Kath described how this altered the RRT worker's practice:

'You've not got so much invested in it. It's a very time-limited, task-specific interaction. Almost like a relationship in a vacuum. It's literally in that moment of time. It doesn't necessarily have to be like that because you could theoretically see someone on duty several times, or it might be someone you worked with once before many years ago. But it often is just that 45-minute space. That's your relationship. So, it's very much a task-centred thing because you've been told: "We're going to do this, or he needs to have a care package or he needs this benefit form filling in" or something. I think you might present as the same nice, friendly person or what have you, but it's a shallower version.'

Consequently, although these remain *relational* spaces of practice, there is a shift in the nature of interpersonal interactions from depth to surface as a result of the temporal constraints, sporadic nature and task-oriented focus of the duty model. Such shifts incur the potential loss of affective dimensions of worker–service user encounters that play a crucial role in generating productive interpersonal connections (Broadhurst and Mason, 2014).

An important example is trust (as discussed in Chapter 3). Kath noted both the importance of and the challenges involved in fostering this quality in short-term duty work:

'I was having a conversation with a client recently. I mean I've only known her about three or four years. 'Only'! Sounds quite a long time to some people, but we were talking about how trust works as a two-way street within the relationship. So, it's not just about them trusting me but me trusting her. So, we were talking about how when she says she'll meet me I can feel reassured that she won't go and harm herself because she has given me her word, and if I say to her "I'll phone you on this day", that contains her. There is a two-way trusting process. It's about two humans coming together, isn't it, and treating each other with that level of respect. So, I think what might've changed is quite often the duty system stops you or doesn't allow for that length of time because you're on once a week or whatever it is and you're seeing different people all the time.'

Leslie also noted that "people who were at risk of really serious relapse, [this had been] prevented and minimised as a consequence of fairly regular, appointments and meaningful relationship with a care coordinator, CPN [community psychiatric nurse] or a social worker".

However, in the RRT, relational spaces are increasingly foreclosed, and these examples highlight the potential losses incurred through a shift from a relationship-based care coordination model towards short-term crisis management. As former CMHT manager Evelyn argued, the opportunities for practitioners to foreground and develop these qualitative dimensions of their work had diminished in the RRT and consequently interventions had become "more about throughput than actual quality of work, more about quantity".

Alongside, and related to, this shift in the balance between the qualitative aspects of care coordination and quantitative pressures of duty work, the greater use of clinics represented another significant manifestation of 'fragmentation through specialisation'. Increasingly, health and care-related practices that might have been delivered individually to service users through the relationship with their care coordinator were organised and delivered centrally through clinics for interventions such as depot injections, health screening, smoking cessation and benefits forms.

Kath explained that for many team members, clinics had been "a bit of an anathema to us. We thought we don't want impersonal clinics where [service users] are queuing up at the door". She considered this emblematic of the overall trend towards "a lot more fragmentation". However, Kath had recently taken on the role of running the RRT's depot clinic, and now she acknowledged some positive aspects:

'If you've got 20 care coordinators, they might not realise that half of their caseload hasn't had their blood pressure taken in the last year. Whereas if you've got one person checking into all the physical health it catches it. But in a way it also dilutes staff work or maybe it specialises it.'

Nonetheless, she saw resource considerations as the primary driver of these changes. "Groups are the most cost-effective way to see clients. Depot clinic is a prime example of that. I'm sat in a room and 30 clients come to me."

There was one other potential area of 'fragmentation through specialisation' that, while not yet implemented, had left RRT social workers feeling that their integrated status within NHS community mental health services was under threat. Social worker Ruth noted a recent local review of the partnership arrangement between the local authority and Trust under which social workers are integrated within NHS mental health services. She explained that the local authority:

'are not happy at all because they pay the Trust a load of money and the Trust are not doing what they should be doing, like, the Care Act assessments, carers assessments. So, there was a big debate about whether we [social workers] should be removed completely. Thankfully they agreed not to do that, but there's still lots of debate about whether to stop us from care coordinating and make sure that we do all the paperwork.'

Partnership agreements have come under pressure across the country in the context of austerity and market reform. Consequently, in some parts of England, social workers have already been withdrawn from integrated mental health teams in order to refocus their work on meeting local authority-specific performance indicators, which are different from those for the NHS (Lilo and Vose, 2016). Ruth's response evokes concern about this potential narrowing of social workers' role in longer-term social-relational work and a concomitant reorientation towards more short-term assessment tasks to meet the local authority's informational demands. Such trends highlight both the wider relationship between labour process fragmentation and the neoliberalisation of funding structures, and the sense that social work's status is increasingly precarious within this setting.

From relational to informational practice

As well as this shifting modality within relational practice, there was also a more general reorientation away from social-relational approaches and towards informational systems in the everyday work of RRT practitioners. Two examples will illustrate this.

As noted earlier, 'clinical zoning' (Ryrie et al, 1997; Adams et al, 2020) had been introduced across the Trust, including at the RRT. Zoning practices emerged in the context of concerns that the Care Programme Approach (CPA) had proven insufficiently dynamic and responsive to changing circumstantial factors in relation to risk (Ashir and Marlowe, 2009). There are a number of elements of a zoning approach. However, this primarily involves the use of a traffic-light system to identify and assess 'clients of concern'. They are then allocated into red, amber and green zones according to perceived levels of risk and need as a means of prioritising team interventions and resources (Adams et al, 2020).

This methodology had been mobilised in various ways in the RRT, most recently in the context of ten-minute 'stand-up' meetings held daily each morning and attended by all RRT team members, in order to assess and manage risk and focus the team and practitioners' interventions accordingly. After initial "mixed feelings", such meetings became, for Kath, "probably a beneficial thing". However, Kath explained that this zoning approach now extended beyond RRT morning meetings and had become an integral feature of the core weekly team meetings. Those meetings were:

'really different to the team meetings we used to have. They're kind of manager-led and risk-led. I mean the [CMHT] meetings, God I remember, they used to go on for several hours and we'd all sit in a big circle and allocate and there would just be a lot of stuff coming up. But now it's like clients of concern and the inpatients and when are they going to be discharged, barriers to discharge, any discharges coming up, any transfers coming up, safeguarding.'

The contrast with the more open and discursive format of weekly meetings at Southville CMHT was stark. As Kath recalled, it was common there to have extended discussions among several team members to explore and share ideas on potential causes of and responses to crisis situations for particular service users. However, the practice in RRT meetings was very different:

'There isn't that open, free-for-all discussion. It's kind of directed to managers and doctors, you know, so we have the clients of concern and it's like: "Oh, I've got this client and his mental state is this, that or the other." Theoretically anyone could chip in and sometimes do but it feels more like it's directed towards doctors, or it's just being documented. So, if something happens, it can be said that we were on it, so more defensive practice. "Here's the plan, you do this, next one." It feels like a management structure. It doesn't feel what we necessarily want to bring up.'

The contrast described by Kath is suggestive of a shift away from CMHT meetings characterised by explorations of service user need and risk based on longitudinal relational engagements. This had been possible because longer-term service users may have been care coordinated by several team members during their time with the service. Instead, in the RRT there was a greater focus on biomedically oriented practices of mental state examination and the associated informational priorities required to defensively manage risk and facilitate throughput. Moreover, this zoning orientation was experienced as enforcing a standardisation and proceduralisation of practice.

Social worker Yvonne described a further application of zoning, implemented during the transition to the RRT. Managers required practitioners to "sort through" all the service users on their caseloads to identify those "who don't really need our team. We're left with people who are in higher need, so we don't really have any more amber, green, they're all red. We don't really have many 'backburner' clients. There is this real push for discharge."

Consequently, clinical zoning was perceived as operating primarily to facilitate service user discharges, a cause for concern among former CMHT practitioners. Yvonne explained that the criteria for such discharge decisions were that "clients have been well for maybe over a year, they're compliant with medications, they've not had an admission in the last three or four years". These examples highlight the imbrication of biological indicators (mental state, medication), risk assessment and resource management in the organisational processes of the RRT. During the CMHT era, the tendency towards *biomedical residualism* was experienced as a pressure bearing on individual practitioners and reshaping elements of relational practice. But now this directional tendency had become more deeply embedded in the organisational structures of the RRT itself.

A second and even more fundamental indicator of the foregrounding of informational practice systems in the RRT was the focus on performance management and 'performative culture' at both individual and institutional levels. A key mechanism through which the Trust and practitioners themselves were able to ascertain their individual-level attainment of organisational key performance indicators (KPIs) was via their computer dashboard. That used a traffic-light system to illustrate the status of individual indicators such as CPA completion and review, risk assessments, HoNOS scores, users' diagnostic, health and demographic data, most recent contact date and so on. Kath explained that:

'[Y]ou access it through the intranet, and you pull up the clinical dashboard and then you can look at yourself and you can look at any of your colleagues, which is always interesting. So, every now and then they'll be like: "Oh you got all green or you've got a lot of red or whatever it might be."'

For Leslie, this visibility and comparability of data generated a disciplining effect, experienced as: "I ought to get mine really up to date. There was a degree of pressure, which is what it was intended to do." The Trust "sent around emails telling teams which were furthest ahead with their targets and outcomes". In this way, the Trust "encouraged the competitive culture" at both individual and team level.

Moreover, the demands of this new informational culture, Yvonne argued, squeezed out the relational aspects of RRT work:

'My worry is, and it has been for some time, that we have more exposure to the computer than we have to therapeutic intervention with our clients, really. The emphasis is more on getting the dashboard completed, that it's green, that we're meeting targets, as opposed to the quality of work that we do with our clients.'

Yvonne evoked a new "management ethos", which she referred to as a "measurement mentality" to capture this tendential shift from qualitative to quantitative considerations.

Leslie also described the marginalisation of social-relational approaches, noting that "appointments become shorter and shorter, in order to prioritise what we were being asked for [targets]". This practice orientation to what is quantified in KPIs (the informational) at the expense of less quantifiable aspects of practice (the relational) is an outcome of a KPI culture that, Smith (1995) argues, leads to 'tunnel vision'.

In spite of these pressures and constraints, Yvonne described how many of the longer-serving practitioners sought to maintain social-relational approaches. However, in this new informational and performative culture, these choices became visible to managers and, consequently, "you find that our dashboard might not look great, we might not have all our plans done because we are putting more input of our time to our clients".

In contrast to these acts of relational recalcitrance, Kath identified how some other practitioners had just aligned to these informational practice systems. "Some people clearly feel the need for it all to be green and that they are seen to be doing their work. But sometimes the people whose dashboards are all green are the ones that actually you think you're not doing very much. I don't really rate what you're doing." Kath, however, resisted this 'green dashboard' orientation, arguing that client care was the important stuff, not "bureaucratic targets". KPI culture has, nonetheless, increasingly reoriented the focus of practice towards the metric itself rather than the underlying objective of reducing service users' mental distress. This is an example of what Smith (1995) terms 'measure fixation'.

An important organisational space for the embedding and inculcation of this shift from social-relational to informational approaches was clinical and professional supervision. Yvonne described how, during the CMHT era, there was a greater orientation towards professional development and support in this setting.

'[However,] supervision now is led by bringing your dashboard out and what needs to be done. And the newer staff, that will be their supervision and that's the culture that they're becoming accustomed to. I think the newer staff, they're being trained that supervision is more around data and stats being important.'

This reflects a broader refocusing of supervision in the context of neoliberal reform of public services in ways that strengthen practitioner instrumentalism in meeting organisational goals, and as a technology of managerial surveillance (Beddoe and Davys, 2016). The tendencies towards generational shifts in terms of the internalisation of performative demands noted by Yvonne can be understood in the context of this new organisational culture.

Another consequence of performance-related pressures was that practitioners' regularly felt no choice but to extend their working day through unpaid overtime to meet these increased informational workload demands and avoid potential disciplinary sanctions from management. CMHN Leslie described the resentment he felt that was generated by the experience of regularly working an additional 15 per cent above his contracted hours because of "deadlines to deliver pieces of work, unrealistic deadlines". In the absence of collective challenges via trade unions and political action, "there was a real recognition among practitioners that this was how things are, but yet no sense of how it might be tackled".

However, Yvonne did note that, sometimes, the purpose of working additional hours was to try to ensure adequate support to service users in the context of resource constraints. The same was true of Kath's efforts to maintain relational engagement in spite of dashboard demands. In these senses, engagement in additional work did not reflect the internalisation of performative demands but might be regarded instead as a form of micro-resistance to neoliberalisation underpinned by a countervailing tendency towards ethico-political professionalism. However, in so far as these acts involved stretching the working day, such ethical orientations functioned to increase the rate of exploitation of workers and thereby subsidise an increasingly residualised mental health system through unpaid labour (Baines, 2004). This ethical stance thus incurred significant emotional and temporal costs for practitioners.

This discussion of dashboard culture highlights the role of performance management and performativity (and its discontents) at the individual level. But Kath also bemoaned the increasing focus on performativity at the institutional level. She described an accentuated and accelerated focus on the demands of informational practice systems in the context of regimes of inspection and regulation. "We've got to suddenly get all the CPAs done in one month. All our risk assessments have to be up to date", because "the CQC's[12] coming round so we have to polish the table". In this sense, the orientation towards a 'green dashboard' is a performative stance underpinning the crafting by senior management of the Trust's public image in order to open up or preserve its funding streams.

Many practitioners noted an increased emphasis by the Trust on these performative aspects of organisational processes. The attendant shift in managerial focus from the lived realities of practice to the informational exigencies that formed the raw materials for this performative recrafting of the NHS Trust generated a significant disconnect between senior managers and frontline practitioners. Social worker Ruth recounted an example when she talked about 'revolving door' (RD) service users. RD, in this sense, refers to the phenomenon of frequent and cyclical readmission to psychiatric inpatient settings experienced by some mental health service users, the reduction of which has been a focus of mental health policy and practice at national and local levels in recent years (Jobling, 2014).

> Ruth (social worker): 'I really could not believe, like, when I was talking to our manager about revolving door and she was saying there is no [RD] and I was like, so what do you class as RD? So, the Trust classes someone who is back in hospital within a month. Well, quite often, it takes three or four weeks to sort out a Mental Health Act assessment, so that's why [ironic laughter], the Trust have got their month. If they upped it to two months, there would be a phenomenal amount of revolving door. And our manager did not understand it, because she had read the [Trust] document that there was no [RD] and she took that as read, she has no ability to think outside the box, she is a complete and utter "yes person" and that's who they employ all the time now.'
>
> Steve (social worker): 'It's a bit like *1984*, what they're saying, because everyone denies it, there's no problem, perfect service.'
>
> Martin (welfare rights): 'It's like if you redefine things, like your revolving door, so if you have to achieve something, rather than actually try and achieve it, you can find the parameters so that you can achieve it, even though you're not really achieving it. So, it's like "new-speak", isn't it? The words used to describe something change the reality.'

Here, the practitioners drew attention to the dissonance between their lived experiences and the performative role of data and statistics articulated by the Trust and defended by the manager. This description is suggestive of what could be termed the 'Performative NHS Trust' (see Jones et al, 2020). This performativity, as noted in Chapter 1, took the form of artificial representations, or 'fabrications' (Ball, 2003) based on metrics, which are crafted by NHS organisations to meet market-oriented managerialist demands in the mental healthcare sector that emanate from the neoliberal state and its array of regulators, auditors and funding bodies. Practitioners frequently expressed exasperation with institutional performativity in the contemporary NHS, particularly when the associated organisational narratives crafted to carefully position the Trust in healthcare markets were felt to be so strongly at odds with the daily experiences of practitioners and their service users.

Furthermore, target culture is characterised by the mutual interdependence not only of processes of quantification and fabrication but those of managerial control. The managerial layer Ruth called "yes people" and Leslie called target-oriented "whipcrackers" enforce this new performance-oriented culture. But they also seek to impose a new neoliberal managerialist 'reality' on practitioners and users. These acts of symbolic violence generate an oppressive Orwellian atmosphere within this service setting (Learmonth, 2005).

The impact of austerity on modalities of practice

While the SLM restructure underpinned significant changes in modalities of practice in the RRT, this was further compounded by the effects of austerity measures. The effects of the austerity agenda contributed to the pressures on RRT workers and impacted on their everyday practices in four ways: inpatient bed reductions; reduced approved mental health professional (AMHP) staffing; social care cuts; and welfare reform.

Significant cuts to inpatient beds in the Trust created frequent bed shortages. Nurse Kath described how managers would then announce that "there's no beds in the Trust. And there'll be this frantic sweep round the wards, who can you discharge?" As a consequence, inpatient admissions were typically of much shorter duration. Social worker Yvonne said: "When I started, people had a lengthy admission. Now there's such a push for discharge that people are being discharged far too early, when they're not fully recovered. So, it becomes like a revolving door admission. As soon as they're admitted, we're talking about discharge."

Kath too described increasing "short-termism" in the inpatient setting. She gave the example of service users being discharged rather than being offered weekend leave, and even in instances where this was offered, "the bed will be used, so even if they go on weekend, they probably come back to a different ward".

Another consequence of bed shortages was an escalation in the use of out-of-area placements (OAPs). At the national level, there was an increase of almost 40 per cent in the number of people sent out of their local area for mental health in-patient treatment between 2014/15 and 2016/17 (BMA, 2017). In response, the government's Mental Health Taskforce (2016) committed to ending OAPs by 2021. And Yvonne noted that, although previously widespread in the Trust, by 2018 "because of cost cutting", OAP use had been reduced locally. Nonetheless, the combination of factors highlighted here undermined the continuity in and quality of inpatient care, with significant detrimental impacts experienced by service users and their families (EHRC, 2017; Trewin, 2017), as well as increasing pressures for practitioners.[13]

Social worker Steve now worked for another NHS mental health Trust in the neighbouring town. He told me that bed shortages had been acute when he was working at Southville CMHT, which was part of Lowertown NHS Trust. However they were even greater in his current Trust, because "they have got the beds, but they sold the beds to places like Lowertown Trust". This use of 'fundraising inpatient beds' reflected the emergence of a market in the context of austerity-related scarcity. This practice was initially stimulated by the implementation of the NHS Foundation Trust model. When Trusts achieved Foundation status, they became independent business units operating in a mental healthcare market. Many Trusts sought to reduce costs by cutting bed numbers. However, when sector-wide NHS bed shortages followed, the sale of 'fundraising' beds offered an opportunity to raise revenue. The adoption of this practice by cash-strapped Trusts was further accelerated in the context of NHS funding constraints under austerity (Moth et al, 2018). This market-oriented practice was one factor, alongside an increase in the use of private sector beds, that underpinned the growth of the use of OAPs noted earlier.

These issues also generated impacts for the AMHP duty service. Suitably qualified RRT practitioners[14] were rostered to work in this service for one day per week. But, Yvonne explained, the number of AMHPs in the RRT was now reduced to three, and "the volume of work is immense". This reflected a wider national trend towards declining AMHP numbers (ADASS, 2018). Furthermore, bed shortages detrimentally affected AMHPs and people being assessed because, following Mental Health Act (MHA) assessments, "clients are being kept in police stations, they're being kept in A&E [Accident & Emergency], above the time that they should do because there isn't a bed". Moreover, the rapid inpatient discharges and subsequent 'revolving door' patterns meant, Yvonne continued, that "on AMHP duty, the same name keeps cropping up again and again and you think, gosh, I assessed this person six months ago".

Related to this was the increasing use of community treatment orders (CTOs) as an alternative to admission, with the agreement of formal CTO criteria a further statutory AMHP role. These cyclical trends, leading to increased MHA assessments and CTO use, further intensified AMHP workloads while negatively impacting service users' experiences. Yvonne described a typical AMHP shift involving hours of preparation on the day before, reading up case notes, then typically two or sometimes more "really mentally and physically draining" MHA assessments on the AMHP duty day itself, and then another day afterwards writing up the MHA paperwork. One AMHP duty day therefore involved, in effect, three days' work. By Yvonne's estimate, these factors combined to produce a doubling of AMHPs' workloads. The "AMHP role used to be an attractive role," Yvonne explained, but she no longer felt this way.

Further austerity-related impacts on the work of RRT practitioners were generated by dramatic social care budget reductions. Yvonne contrasted the early days of personalisation with the current austerity era. Then "there was a full pot of money, but that pot of money is completely dissolved now". There had already been "huge pressure" on workers generated by the bureaucratic demands of a 25-page social care funding form for local authority services (for example, homecare, day services and so on), annual re-application and a separate form required for each resource requested. All that "had a huge impact on our workload". But, in addition, practitioners were now increasingly required to attend a panel of social care managers in person to make the case for their funding application. This could be an extremely difficult experience, Yvonne explained, because of the emphasis on spending controls and the hostile atmosphere created to impose this agenda. "Practitioners have left there crying. People have refused to go back to panel because of how they've been treated." Yvonne described the sense of resentment towards local authority management that this created. However, she continued: "[U]ltimately the client needs come first. Although a panel is an awful experience, if a client requires a service and there's essential needs, you have to do it."

One further and final austerity-related issue was welfare reform. This impacted the RRT locally through a cut from three to two welfare rights worker posts within the Trust's community services. Martin explained that the three welfare rights workers were funded by the local authority, and the cut had been absorbed through him and one other colleague mutually agreeing to reduce from a full-time to a part-time post. This meant, compared with the CMHT, he now had fewer hours with which to cover a larger population of RRT service users. Martin said scathingly: "[I]t shows what value they place on the work I'm doing here." The reduced hours meant he was no longer able to support service users with initial benefit applications, only later-stage reconsiderations and appeals. In the past, intervening at the earlier stage had meant he had "managed to avoid people having to attend these awful benefits assessments. Now I can't do preventative. It's a bit like how the health service is generally moving from a preventative to a crisis response. In a way I've followed that movement."

For service users, Martin explained, benefits assessment processes were increasingly harsh and "distressing ... When they've described in detail how difficult and stressful everything is and how everything is a struggle and then they get turned down. It's that feeling of not being believed or not being accepted. That is definitely how the system works." Moreover, the increased delays and more frequent rejections of applications meant users "experience financial hardship. They get really stressed out, they get really agitated, they get really worried. It's very stressful and very difficult. And for some people it can precipitate relapses."

Kath, too, noted the mental health impact of this policy agenda on service users. "It's a massive fear for clients. They're much more anxious." An expanding body of evidence has identified the harms and structural violence associated with this draconian welfare reform agenda, generating high levels of 'benefits distress' for claimants in the process (Moth and Lavalette, 2017; Moth, forthcoming b).

These policy reforms consequently had significant implications for practitioners. As a result of his reduced hours and increased workload pressures, Martin was unable to support service users with initial claims. That work was now "devolving more on other practitioners, care coordinators, a lot of duty is now dealing with benefits stuff as well". Kath described the impact on RRT practitioners:

'We're filling in the forms. Take clients to assessments, you have to write supporting letters, you have to get advice yourself [on benefits rules], phone calls. It's more, it's much more of it. The whole benefits system now is much more punitive isn't it, so it's harder. So, we have to fight more, so you have to devote more energy to it.'

However, during a period that saw a substantial reduction in welfare rights support, the Trust had overseen the addition of dedicated employment support workers across its services. One of these employment support workers, Giles, was based in the RRT. There were a range of responses from practitioners to this role. Kath said she had not really engaged with Giles. Yvonne had recently met with him and identified three service users to refer. Martin felt Giles was "very good at his job", but he was much more ambivalent about this role in general. He noted that Giles was "not pushing people too much" to get work, although this was not necessarily true of other employment support workers.

Martin was not happy with this refocusing of resources away from welfare rights and towards employment support. "Work makes you free I think it's called, or something,"[15] Martin said, and gave an angry laugh. "That's coming through the benefits system as well," he added. "That's definitely a big push these days." This highlights both the workfare focus within the contemporary neoliberal welfare state, which Friedli and Stearn (2015) term 'psychocompulsion', and an increasing alignment of neoliberal healthcare policy goals with this workfare agenda, visible for instance in the discourse of 'employment as a health outcome' articulated within the *Five Year Forward View for Mental Health* (Moth and McKeown, 2016; McKenna et al, 2019).

Overall, these changes to modalities of practice in the RRT reflect a deepening of all four dimensions of strenuous welfarism described in Chapter 2. Developments such as the standardisation of risk assessment through clinical zoning practices reflect the codification of practitioners' knowledge to enable more comprehensive audit and control. The intensification of worker effort was visible in, and facilitated by, the increased orientation to informational practices and 'dashboard culture' in the RRT. These increased administrative burdens led to further reductions in time for relational support to service users. At the organisational level of the RRT this was reflected in a shifting balance towards short-term duty work rather than care coordination. Finally, a loss of breathing space and porous time was reflected in what Kath described as the increasingly 'quiet' offices of the RRT where reflective case discussions and social interactions between practitioners were increasingly marginalised in order to deliver conditions for greater informational productivity. The combination of these various aspects of strenuous welfarism meant that, for CMHN Kath, "teams have been stretched and stretched until now they've lost all elasticity".

Shifting temporalities of practice

This section will focus on the accelerating tempos and rhythms associated with the changing modalities of practice. The first, *constraints on time for social-relational approaches*, was described by participants as endemic in the RRT in the context of escalating requirements to complete informational tasks.

Leslie had "less time to focus on supporting people to identify their strengths and their abilities, in order to identify some aspirations that they might have to work more towards. A lot of that work was cut." At the CMHT, as we saw earlier, Leslie had implemented a strengths-based approach through tools such as the 'tree of life' from narrative therapy. But in spite of his efforts to maintain some focus on this type of strengths-based work, "that ended up just being absolutely not a priority". Nurse Kath used the phrase "hit and run" for the increasingly short face-to-face meetings with service users. The violent imagery suggests the structural harm that such a practice modality involves.

In addition to less time for relational work and shorter appointments, a second temporal shift was the *shorter duration of service provision*, visible in both community and inpatient spheres of service provision. This manifested in the greater focus on brief interventions, throughput and the rapid discharge of service users. This accompanied the shift from long-term care coordination to short-term duty work. Kath evoked these accelerated work rhythms: "Get the work done, move on to the next thing, got to hit the targets." And that, as she explained earlier, led to shallow work.

Welfare rights worker Martin's unique vantage point within but also alongside the team enabled him, too, to discern these new 'throughput' temporalities of casework. "The old-school thing about seeing service users regularly and supporting them and doing things gradually. [Now] it's quicker, more throughput. 'What are you doing with this person? If you're not doing anything, why do they need to be on care coordination?'"

In contrast to this increased tempo and flow of users through services, was the stasis of *institutional waiting*. One example, already raised by social worker Yvonne, was the use of duty as a "holding ground" for service users awaiting allocation for care coordination. Another, also noted by Yvonne, was the wait to receive therapies from the RRT's clinical psychologists. She described how initial assessments for therapy were "fairly quick". But then there was:

'a long wait, maybe about three months, until the client is seen again. During that time, the situations change, clients become more unwell. That's its downfall at the moment, it's the waiting time from the initial assessment when the client feels, "great, I'm being seen" then to be told, "well, you've got a three-month wait".'

These experiences of 'chronic waiting' (Jeffrey, 2008) are potentially harmful, and increasingly common in the context of austerity. While this contradictory nexus of waiting and rapid transitions might seem paradoxical, both phenomena are emergent features of the neoliberalisation of welfare (Soldatic, 2013; McWade, 2015).

A fourth temporal shift relates to mental health workers' own employment trajectories. Their expectations of long-term careers were undermined by changes in both the conditions and nature of work. These trends towards *foreshortened careers* were apparent in the contrast between Evelyn, Roger and Kath, who had all worked in the Trust and its forerunners since qualifying as nurses, and Leslie who had left the Trust in 2014 after 25 years' working in NHS secondary mental health services. Leslie explained that he had found himself deeply unsatisfied with a role in an RRT dominated by "crunching numbers in front of a PC". For similar reasons, Yvonne was questioning whether she could continue in her social work post after 17 years' service. Ruth noted that the average career span of a social worker was now only seven years due to workload pressures and burnout (Baginsky, 2013; Ravalier, 2019).

Kath believed that "new nurses coming into [the role] are not going to have a 30-year stint, five to ten years maybe because they're just being spat out, chewed up by the system". These foreshortened career spans were problematic for many reasons. But for Kath, a particular issue was the importance of practitioners' role in "holding histories". Initially, she related this to knowledge of service users' histories and experiences, in particular "bearing witness" to their lived experiences as a form of interpersonal validation and therapeutic support. However, she later extended this to include an organisational dimension. "There's four of us left that are holding that history and we remember the 'Walk-In'[16] and we bring it up, whereas all the new staff they had no sense of, that that's a facility that could be there." This institutional history enables alternative horizons of possibility that reach beyond individualised and market-oriented forms of provision based on eligibility criteria and extend more holistically towards wider communities.

Countervailing responses to temporal shifts

While, as this chapter so far has highlighted, there are prominent tendencies towards increasing velocities of practice and provision within the RRT, temporal processes and experiences in this context are nonetheless differentiated. Human agency and resistance intervene (Rosa, 2017; Vostal et al, 2019). A dominant institutional temporality, generated by subsumption (see Chapter 8) and associated market mechanisms, manifests in the rhythmic acceleration of informational accountability and throughput. However, alternative institutional and disciplinary temporalities, associated with social-relational, therapeutic or biomedical ideas and practices, are also visible.

A further temporal layer is the experiential, which articulates subjective dimensions of temporality. For workers, the intentional and contingent flows of temporal experience within labour processes may manifest as movement between accelerated juggling of tasks and, more rarely, slowing to reflect on a situation. Mental health service users' experiential temporality may encompass waiting and wasting, aspiration and hope (McWade, 2015).

These diverse temporalities may sometimes align, at others collide, producing frictions at the intersections of temporal orders that are 'out of sync'. The temporal agency of workers and service users in the field is visible as they synchronise between, adapt and accommodate to and subvert (or resist) these different temporalities in their everyday practices of producing mental health work.

There were a number of examples of such temporal agency in the RRT. The first relates to processes of 'fragmentation through specialisation' outlined earlier, in this case the expansion of the clinic model. Kath's manager had asked her to run the depot (long-acting injection) clinic at the RRT. At first, Kath had reservations. Clinics had not been a feature at Southville CMHT due to the widely held perception of them as "impersonal", evoking queues of service users at the door. Kath eventually agreed to this role but was clear that she "didn't want it to feel like a white coat clinic". Instead, she explained:

> 'I've been very clear that I want a really relaxed depot clinic. So there's a lot of banter and it's not, you know, it's very low-key assessment, you know, if there is any assessment at all. I'm not going to be looking at mood states and things like that. And some of the clients it's, it can be really nice and relaxed. So I'm always sort of chatting to people.'

Her hope was that "there is a continuity, so I get to know all the clients and they get to know me". In this way, Kath had sought to achieve a temporal reordering of the clinic as a 'relaxed' space for dialogical interpersonal interactions, rather than simply a rapid and depersonalised production line of biomedical interventions. She did so by asserting temporal agency in the form of an intentional slowdown of practice in order to foster these social-relational engagements.

She was challenging the dominant institutional temporality within which the clinic functions as a mechanism for delivering cost efficiencies. After all, depot injections could potentially be delivered in a matter of seconds. Thus, in spite of her earlier misgivings: "In truth, I quite like the depot clinic because I think part of the joys of this work is that kind of taking ownership, control, responsibility of your work as opposed to being told and monitored." Kath's intervention constituted a form of micro-resistance or ethico-political praxis.

A second example highlights emergent tensions between the dominant throughput model and professional temporalities associated with community mental health nursing and social work that have historically foregrounded more temporally extended forms of relationship-based practice and therapeutic engagements. Frictions and opposition to this institutional shift arose among some practitioners (and service users) because, as Kath explained, "our expectations were longer-term work. Discharge was not something that was pushed or a frequent occurrence. It happened and it was quite a big event."

Leslie described responding to this discharge-focused approach in the RRT by "just trying to use my experience to protect, as much as I could, people on the caseload, if you like, to drag my heels a bit about discharge and to try and work around the system as best I could really for those clients". However, this exertion of temporal agency to 'slow down' discharges, and enable ongoing therapeutic support, was only temporarily effective. When Leslie left, the service was withdrawn from many long-term users, often with, he speculated, deeply harmful consequences. Nonetheless, Leslie had asserted temporal agency as a form of resistance to demands for institutional 'throughput'.

A third instance of temporal agency relates to efforts to 'hold histories' in opposition to dominant neoliberal discourses of dependency creation directed at long-term mental health work (Raco, 2009; Slade, 2009; Collins, 2019). Evelyn directly addressed the notion that relational forms of professional practice in the earlier CMHT era were necessarily static and fostered service dependency,

'The whole ethos and culture at that time was, yes, we had our own pressure to discharge people because we didn't want to create that dependency on services. And we wanted people to be able to do as much as possible that they could, you know, so it wasn't that we were wanting to hold onto people. So, there was all those kinds of checks and balances. It's like a support network, which was tight at one end maybe and then just loosened and loosened and loosened. But nobody was ever kind of cast off, unless it was absolutely clear that, you know, [the] GP was up for it, the client was up for it and that there was never any problem about coming back.'

For Evelyn, this carefully managed gradualism was consistent with the longstanding disciplinary temporalities of nursing and social work. These recognised the fluctuating, unpredictable and sometimes extended temporalities of mental distress. It was therefore possible to adjust the tempos and intensity of therapeutic work accordingly.

However, these capacities for temporal flexibility have been significantly eroded. Nonetheless, progressive 'archaic remnants' (Harootunian, 2015) also endured in the practice of longstanding team members such as Yvonne and Kath, who continue to 'hold the histories' of the remaining longer-term service users on their caseload while also attempting to orient to social-relational interventions and ethico-political and rights-based practices wherever possible.

This chapter has outlined three major structural changes impacting on service provision since the first phase of the study. These are: the austerity agenda; welfare reform; and the SLM reorganisation that created RRTs. The SLM model accelerates service commodification processes by extending the quantification of units of provision via service lines (care pathways). The earlier CMHT model was dominated by more indeterminate, relational modes of work (Harrison, 2009), although this was being eroded, whereas the informational practice system to record and measure activity is an integral and requisite feature of the newer marketised structures of the RRT. However, the interaction between SLM reforms and austerity-related retrenchment has generated significant tensions and constraints, which have been experienced at multiple levels including the temporal. The chapter has drawn attention to frictions generated at the intersection between colliding temporalities, but also forms of temporal agency and resistance.

Shifting contours of managerial control

The previous chapter provided an overview of the Rehabilitation and Recovery Team (RRT) model that superseded the Community Mental Health Team (CMHT). The RRT represented an evolution of NHS institutional structures that more firmly embedded neoliberal priorities and forms of control in its organisational design. However, institutional reforms such as this should always be understood as the outcome of interactions between agents shaped by particular conditions of sociostructural possibility.

This chapter gives a more granular picture of forms of agency in this setting. There are three parts to the chapter. First, nurse and trade union activist Roger offers an overview of the shifting landscape of relations between trade unions and senior managers from the latter stages of the community care era up until the RRT restructure. Second, the disciplining and victimisation of team manager Evelyn provides a case study of intensified processes of managerial control during this period. The third section then examines how Roger, Evelyn and other practitioners responded, both individually and collectively, to these organisational reforms and shifting frontiers of control.

Shifting frontiers of control in statutory mental health services

Power and conflict in the labour process: Roger's perspective

We begin with Roger, who was a leading figure in organising a strike by mental health nurses in 1992, when he and his colleagues were employed by the local health authority, the forerunner of the current NHS Trust. Roger recalled this experience fondly: "It was just wonderful."

He explained that the dispute had arisen after two senior managers had come to a weekly meeting of mental health nurses from across the health authority. The managers announced that "they'd been looking at the way staffing was organised and said there was going to be a new way of working, a thing called 'skills mix', which basically was about [staffing] cuts". Furthermore, the four nurses whose posts were earmarked to be cut were all from racialised communities or non-British nationality backgrounds. Some other posts were also downgraded, meaning salary reductions. Roger described the mood of shock in the room after the managers left. "We couldn't believe it, nobody could take it in." One of the senior nurses present, who was also an active trade unionist, turned to those gathered and said: "If you're worried about it then you've got to do something about it. You are the G grade [senior nurses]. You don't realise how powerful you are." Then, "we sort of got organised," Roger said.

Sharon, another mental health nurse, and Roger were the local representatives for the Confederation of Health Service Employees (COHSE)[1] trade union at their respective workplaces. For Roger, this was the day hospital then located on the Southville site. Sharon was based at a larger inpatient unit. Roger and Sharon took the lead in building support in each location, recruiting numerous new union representatives in the process. Meanwhile, the union's regional officer wrote to senior management to challenge both the discriminatory nature of the cuts and the lack of consultation. Management refused to negotiate. So, Roger explained, the union called a day of strike action. Roger had valuable experience from the 1988 national nurses' strike, which had won significant pay increases for nurses (Hayward and Fee, 1992; Fagan, 2013). He drew on that to inform organising of this more localised action four years later.

The strike happened on a wintery Friday in February. Approximately 100 mental health nurses were covered by the dispute. "Over 90 were rostered in and didn't go to work. It was just fully supported, it was great," Roger recounted. Rallies on the day were visited by local Members of Parliament (MPs) and "people from the [local general hospital] came out [in support] in their lunch breaks. The best thing was it didn't rain, but it was a bit chilly!" The strike was even aided by solidarity from some Royal College of Nursing (RCN) members who, at that time, had a no-strike policy.[2] Roger recalled one higher grade nurse who said: "What you're doing is right. Because I'm in the RCN I can't strike, but I will make sure I will work that day. I will be the senior on call, so no COHSE members have to go [in]." Organising emergency ward cover in this way enabled the maximum number of COHSE members to join the strike.

Roger described eagerly waiting for news the following Monday morning, and soon the union representatives got word that a meeting had been called by management for Thursday. Roger, Sharon and the representatives were joined by the COHSE regional officer for the meeting. Management had "never met anybody quite like him," Roger said of the officer. "He had a lot of experience." Filing into the room, the reps "sat on opposite sides of a table" from the senior managers. Management "had these proposals and so [the regional officer] said 'OK, what are they?' Anyway, they went through them, they didn't want repetition [of the strike], but it was hard to take in." Having heard the proposals, the COHSE officer called an adjournment to the meeting. After management representatives had left the room the officer said: "We've done it! Have you seen what they said there? They just basically went back on everything. It was back to the status quo."

The major concession of reversing the proposed staffing and pay cuts was point three on the senior managers' list. It had been blandly worded and sandwiched between a number of other less pertinent points so that Roger and others had barely registered it. The union representatives sought clarification on this issue once the managers returned to the room, and they confirmed it. "So we'd stopped them," Roger said gleefully. The consequence was that lots of the senior managers involved "left with their tails between their legs. Yeah, they were out of the organisation. I think they were encouraged" to leave.

For Roger, this comprehensive victory not only had immediate benefits, shifting the balance of power from management to unions, but also left a significant legacy for the next decade or so. He detailed these effects. "While this was going on there were places cutting everywhere throughout and our aim was to make sure that we didn't get any cuts. So, that's why for a long time" nurses in this health authority "always were on a grade higher than anyone else in the country. Yeah, after '92, because of the strike we held back the cuts." Roger explained that the new director of nursing, who joined shortly after the strike, signalled he wanted "better communication between staff side and management, jaw jaw rather than war war. They were shit scared we were going to go out on strike [again]."

Roger reflected on mental health nurses' motivations for joining the strike. "It was a real mixture. [For] some it was just about their pockets [pay] but there were some who it was about the impact on services and that patients would get a worse, that it wouldn't be such a good deal for them. And there'd be less [professional] expertise around" due to cuts. Roger identified with the latter more overtly ethical and political orientation among some practitioners. He was critical of service reforms that meant service users had "less time with staff. I wanted to be paid properly but it wasn't the be all and end all. I quite enjoyed what I was doing and there was an element of 'patients first'. That was always my sort of approach." He talked about empathy with service users. "I was just glad I wasn't in that system, and I have my moments" in terms of mental health. Roger summed up this ethos in his oft-used phrase "diagnosis human", which he deployed to contrast his own ethical stance with a dehumanising biomedical reductionism in some strands of psychiatry.

These instances of successful collective action built political confidence among nurses to continue to challenge management for improved conditions until the mid-1990s. As Roger put it, "done it once, just do it again". However, some of the minor 'skills mix' concessions granted by the union in 1992, for instance devolving responsibilities such as emergency on-call cover to less experienced staff, began to incrementally expand from the late 1990s. Moreover, across the next decade, Roger described a decline in union activity, with recruitment to the union becoming harder. "Far less people wanted to rock the boat." That was partly because of "what Thatcherism did to people". However, he also felt the 1993 merger of the health unions into UNISON, a larger but more diffuse organisation, contributed to this trend. With the reorganisation of health authorities into NHS Trusts under the New Labour government in 2002, and then national reforms to NHS pay and conditions structures as part of Agenda for Change in 2004, pay improvements established through industrial action during the 1980s and 1990s were eroded.

These trends were, moreover, significantly reinforced by the granting of 'Foundation' status to the NHS Trust in 2008, which meant the organisation became a relatively independent business unit. "As soon as the [Foundation] Trust was coming in they found ways of saving money, which was axing staff and also taking away terms and conditions." One of these ways was the ending of five-year salary protection for staff in the event of redeployment, an increasingly common experience in a context of frequent service reconfigurations. Roger described his response when this plan was announced at a management–union joint negotiating meeting with Trust senior management:

'I actually got them to repeat themselves, I remember being very basic about it: "So I started in 1976, for all that time I've had a protected salary of five years should I have been downgraded and you're saying that won't hold good anymore and it will be down to two years?" So, I said, "Is that what you're saying?" And they said: "Well yeah, we are." And I just said, "You should be absolutely ashamed of yourselves." And none of them could look at me, they just hung their head and looked at the floor, none of them could say anything.'

For Roger, this represented "the final straw", the culmination of incremental shifts in the balance of power from the trade union to senior management within the Trust and its predecessors since the 1990s. In his view this constrained the scope for unions to contest New Public Management (NPM) reforms implemented through organisational reconfigurations, redesigned skills mix divisions of labour, and adjustments to pay and conditions. As a result of these changes, "the staff-side unions were just decimated". Trust senior management "didn't want a staff-side [union] after that, they just said: 'We can do what we want, we don't need it.'"

Although significant in terms of union organising, these changes were just one element of shifting power relations within statutory mental health services. With the establishment of NHS Foundation Trusts, accountability mechanisms such as elected governors were introduced. Union activists sought to exert some influence on Trust policy through this process, and UNISON trade union colleagues persuaded Roger to stand as a 'staff governor' representative. "I was encouraged to do that, the red under the bed so to speak!" However, when Roger was elected and began attending the Trust Board, "it became very apparent that, … whenever we used to have these meetings", any staff representative who spoke, management "would just ignore us. But anything a patient said they would be alert, and, 'Oh yeah, we must do something about that, we hear what you're saying.'"

This highlights the structural influence of service user involvement, which began to become increasingly prominent in statutory services from the late 1990s onwards. By chance, two of the service user governor representatives were people Roger was acquainted with as they had used services at Southville. Roger noted that: "These two absolutely hated [management], more than I did actually!" So a dialogue began to develop between these service user representatives and Roger. It "was unofficial, informal chats about things". These discussions typically focused on coordinating questions to ask at Board meetings, but they also talked about proposed service cuts and closures.

One instance was the announcement in 2008 of the Trust's plan to close the Walk-In service based at Southville. Roger described public consultation meetings, covered in the local press, at which Trust senior managers were berated by irate service users who valued the Walk-In. Roger recalled that Ken, the Trust director of social care, "was there for a bit and he did his stuff because he was one of those who were trying to institute it. And then when he left [the consultation meeting] I thought well, I best show him out and he said: 'I can't believe how angry [the service users] are.' I said, 'don't you realise, this is fundamental. It is a loss, they are going to be angry, upset and depressed about it. It's basic, if you look at the clinical stuff to do with mental health, losses are significant'". Roger paused. "I never got on with him, he just couldn't even see it was going to be a loss."

There is a stark contrast, for Roger, between this senior manager's disregard for service users' collective concerns about the closure and his own sense of empathy and solidarity with the service users' position. An orientation towards solidarity with service users was often in evidence among other Southville practitioners too. Furthermore, Roger's recollections foreground nascent informal collaborations between trade union and service user representatives within the Trust. However, more formal activist interventions and sustained joint campaigning by workers alongside service users, did not emerge during the fieldwork. The restrictive trade union legislation noted earlier was a barrier to deepened solidarity, as well as constraining notions of service user–professional boundaries in mental health services that problematise such activities. So too were differing political and ethical stances among practitioners. Nonetheless, some of the foundations for 'Sedgwickian' service user–worker alliances oriented to more democratic services (Sedgwick, 2015) were clearly visible in embryonic form in the co-organising around the Trust Board and the challenge to the Walk-In closure.

The intensification of senior management control: Evelyn's perspective

The shifting power balance between senior management and trade unions at the health authority and then the Trust from the 1980s to 2000s had many significant consequences for the day-to-day experiences of staff and service users. A particularly important element was the role of this struggle in determining the contours of managerial control, and thereby shaping the nature and extent of neoliberal reform implementation (Worrall et al, 2010). Alongside the imposition of the new 'skills mix' divisions of labour and associated roles and bandings within services noted in Chapter 2, reforms also involved the intensification of reconfigured work processes. These sought to embed informational practice with a particular focus on digitalisation via information and communication technology (ICT). Because revenue streams for Foundation Trusts, now independent business units in the NHS market, are linked to meeting ICT-mediated key performance indicators (KPIs), these targets have become an existential preoccupation for Trusts. In this section, I will explore the implications of this new market and target-oriented reality for Evelyn.

The major reorganisation of services in 2012 restructured teams to align with the new funding-oriented service-line management (SLM) system. At that point, six community teams were combined into two RRTs, and a restructure reduced the number of managers. Such cost-saving reductions in management, as well as workers, reflect a common trend in the contemporary National Health Service (NHS) (Hyde et al, 2016). Consequently, those CMHT managers retaining their posts in the new configuration took on more senior managerial responsibilities, while RRT deputy managers were left with more direct responsibility for day-to-day management of each RRT. Evelyn described how the Trust manoeuvred her "out of even being in the pot of people being able to apply" for an RRT manager job. She felt a "great sense of disappointment" about this, even though she had been offered an alternative role as a trainer.

> 'One of the reasons that I was moved out or aside was because they did not like my style of management. [It] just didn't fit with the new system. [The Trust] didn't like the fact that I didn't take on board the kind of task-management, target-driven service that it was turning into. I prioritised clinical care and the management of staff and, you know, management support, supervision of staff, over getting returns done. That's really what they tried to get me on in terms of my disciplinary.'

This disciplinary process had been instigated in the aftermath of a homicide committed by a service user of Southville CMHT. For Evelyn, these events were "a tragedy, but it was used [as] a bit of a witch hunt for the clinician [care coordinator] and myself". This was based on alleged informational gaps at the CMHT, for instance in the recording of risk assessments. Evelyn's disciplinary, she explained, "wasn't technically linked to the homicide". But the issue of recording had been raised, so the Trust "did a big kind of audit". "They trawled through the clinician's records" and then looked at all the informational systems for the whole team.

As a result, the following year, the Trust brought forward 12 charges against Evelyn concerning matters such as the team's sickness and flexible working hours records, "team management, allocation of resources, keeping up to date with records, it was anything. You can imagine, as a practitioner, if you've got your case files, that if somebody comes and wants to find fault with them, they can say, 'but you've got a date of birth there that's wrong.' They trawled through everything, and they chucked everything and anything that they could to make it stick."

The Trust argued that these informational concerns constituted gross misconduct for which Evelyn potentially faced dismissal. The seriousness of the charge, in her view, reflected a "damage limitation" exercise by the Trust.

'To me and my union rep, [the Trust] were going to go for the harshest penalty so that if anything came out of the [homicide] investigations, they would say: "That's the person who's culpable and look what we've done, we've investigated and we've sacked her." Ultimately, in contrast to the Trust's internal investigation, the outcome of an external inquiry into the homicide was that "a lot was blamed on the system [in the Trust] and that it wasn't specific to me and [the care coordinator]".'

Evelyn had already taken out a counter grievance against the Trust, and eventually received a financial settlement in return for dropping her case against it. However, after more than 30 years as a highly regarded practitioner within the health authority and then the Trust, Evelyn experienced the perceived damage to her reputation generated by the disciplinary process as a heavy emotional burden. "It was horrible, it was really, really sad. A number of people knew about the incident, about the disciplinary action and so it was almost like: 'Oh, she must have done something wrong.' It was like, no smoke without fire and so it was the most awful way to leave."

This meant there was no formal Trust-organised retirement celebration to acknowledge her long service to the organisation as was usual practice. Evelyn described her feelings when a party was organised the following year to mark the retirement of another nurse, a friend of Evelyn's with a similar length of service in the Trust. "It was all still a bit raw. It was so hurtful that everything was taken, nothing was proven."

Reflecting on this experience, Evelyn felt there were three "different agendas … all at the same time" that explained why, in her view, she had been "scapegoated" by the Trust. These were that there was somebody to blame in relation to the homicide, that they could save money on a redundancy payment and that "her attitude towards management just is never going to change, so the sooner she goes the better".

For Evelyn, one particularly bitter irony was that the post-CMHT role she had been offered within the Trust was focused on providing risk assessment training to practitioners. When delivering this, she had been required to emphasise the Trust's 'no blame' policy when seeking to understand risk-related incidents. Evelyn's descriptions of her treatment by senior management within the Foundation Trust at this point evoke an authoritarian atmosphere, and a culture of bullying, blame and fear.[3] She described how other practitioners were "hounded out" of their posts in the wake of the restructure.

However, for Roger and Evelyn, one of the ways in which the concerns and criticisms of longstanding practitioners were contained and silenced was through the fear of risks to pension entitlements. For instance, Roger described recounting his criticism of the Trust senior managers at the management-union joint negotiating committee meeting to a trade unionist friend:

'[The friend] told me that I had 18 months, two years to go [before retirement], not to get too involved because, he had some stories of people being sacked for absurd things at [another hospital]. He said they'll find a way of doing it with you and you'll lose all your pension so it's just not worth it.'

Evelyn independently described a similar concern during her grievance procedure against the Trust. She described hearing "all sorts of horror stories" from her union representative. They "were saying: 'They can sack, dismiss, you've got to watch your pension.'" Consequently, she was persuaded to settle early rather than continue her challenge. Moreover, the counsel received by both Roger and Evelyn suggests a culture of fear that extends well beyond this individual Trust management.

Roger and Evelyn's stories illustrate a shift in the frontier of control in the public sector as power shifted from workers and their collective organisations to senior management. The narratives present the period up to early 1990s as characterised by more distributed and collegial forms of control associated with the professional bureaucracies of the Keynesian era, alongside higher levels of worker militancy and trade union influence over workplace conditions. While not obfuscating conflicting worker and manager structural interests during this earlier period, they nonetheless evoke a somewhat more horizontal distribution of power between frontline mental health workers and senior managers, generated by higher levels of struggle and its legacies. However, with the implementation of neoliberal reforms in the organisation and delivery of health and social care from the 1990s onwards, forms of control that were more top down, centralised and coercive became increasingly prominent. These reforms introduced NPM mechanisms in the form of performance management systems to reshape the labour process and realise 'efficiencies' (Worrall et al, 2010). Implementing this neoliberal NPM reform of the labour process necessitated the minimisation and marginalisation of trade union influence in public sector services, including within mental health services.

However, formal trade union resistance to this programme of reforms was relatively limited. There were some small-scale examples of resistance led by local trade union branches and frontline practitioner trade unionists, such as a 2007 strike by NHS workers in Manchester against the NPM reorganisation of mental health services and associated redundancies and cuts (Barker, 2008; McKeown, 2009). However, from the 1990s onwards, the leaderships of the NHS and social services trade unions at the national level accepted the weakening of safeguards to workers' rights and conditions (Ironside and Seifert, 2004, p 68). This reflected escalating legal constraints on trade union activity implemented by neoliberal governments from the 1980s onwards, but also the twin barriers of high levels of bureaucratic inertia by trade union leaderships and relatively low levels of confidence among frontline union members to organise action independently from below (Darlington and Upchurch, 2012). The segmented nature of trade union membership among health and social care workers was another limiting factor. A significant potential obstacle to neoliberal public sector reform in the form of trade union resistance was thus increasingly marginalised, a much more vertical distribution of power emerged and the pace of NPM reforms accelerated (Worrall et al, 2010).

Responding to shifting frontiers of control: institutional role action and collective agency

An important strategic dimension of, and necessity for, the wider neoliberal project since the 1980s has been confrontation with organised labour. The aim was to impose constraints on trade union power and thereby create the conditions for market-oriented institutional restructuring (Mathers et al, 2018). The preceding section has described how this manifested in the mental health system, with a series of incremental neoliberalising reforms implemented by senior managers in a context of the reluctance of bureaucratically oriented trade union leaderships to foster or support collective action. This (contingent) decline in trade union activity and a concomitant increase in the concentration of institutional control in the hands of senior managers enabled a realignment of the core activities of mental health services with new market-oriented priorities.

Emergentist Marxism's account of agency, briefly outlined in Chapter 1,[4] is based on a stratified model of people, where practitioners are understood as institutional role actors, socialised into adherence to particular professional norms, theoretical systems and forms of action. But equally they are also understood as social agents, through their social positioning within the allocative and authoritative resource distributions of capitalism. The latter pre-structure their positional interests in society and generate an attendant potential for collective forms of agency, for example trade union activity. Consequently, the activity of mental health workers is shaped *both* by their institutional role as, for instance, social worker or nurse, *and* by social agency in so far as they participate in collectivities such as labour or social movements.[5] These identifications matter because they influence how people make sense of and respond organisationally and politically to the circumstances within which they find themselves (Creaven, 2000).

The influence of, and fluctuations between, these identities were apparent in some of the rationales given by practitioners for the changing organisational structures and managerial regimes they encountered. For instance, both Evelyn and Roger evoked the new culture associated with health and social care integration when articulating concerns about oppressive senior managerial practices. Evelyn's direct line manager, who coordinated her disciplinary, was from a local authority background and, in her view, this shaped his approach. Consequently, she argued, while he "was part of the Trust he was still steeped in social services". Unlike the NHS, this "was a different culture: you do as you're told, there's no argument with it". Roger, too, sometimes referred in frustration to "bloody social services". He considered problematic managerial practices in NHS mental health services to have arisen, at least in part, from local authority–NHS organisational integration since the 1990s.

While some used this lens of interagency cultural differences arising from health and social services integration, others used a prism of interprofessional competition and social closure[6] to explain the organisational constraints on professional practice. For instance, a narrative of declining status and influence for their respective professional groups was articulated by both consultant psychiatrist James as well as Evelyn. Their point of comparison was with clinical psychology, which had, they both separately argued, succeeded in strengthening its position within this evolving institutional domain. For James, psychiatry's current intellectual status compared unfavourably with the dynamism of contemporary psychology, and this underpinned the latter's challenge to psychiatry's leading position within the mental health field.

The various orientations suggest that these practitioners' frame of analysis was shaped by their positioning within a system of institutional role action.

In all these instances, however, the practitioners' positioning was not static. When James later reflected on these professional and organisational processes and the tensions and contradictions created by them, he sought to distance himself from his earlier comments about psychology. He offered an alternative reading, arguing that the horizontal divisions between occupational groupings exacerbated by professional defensiveness in a context of neoliberal managerialism and austerity are better understood as an expression of vertical socioeconomic power differentials. James was self-critical, noting that he had constructed the relationship "in a very tribalistic way".

'"It's us and them, we had the power, we lost it, now they've got it." But actually, it's an illusion anyway … The way power is shared around in the health service, these aren't horizontal divisions, it's not this profession or that profession, it's bosses and workers. Maybe it becomes more, you know, more emphasised in a time of recession, rather than in a time of expansion. So I don't know, I suppose, to some extent, the health service has expanded in some ways after '97 and it's retracting now. And so, you know, in those circumstances, the actions of bosses are more likely to come into conflict with the interests of workers.'

James reflected on the reasons for this 'tribalism':

'I'd over-identified with psychiatry or psychiatrists as a, with an identity, as a grouping, as kin. And I think that was a kind of entrenched or defensive retreat, in the face of, you know, the barrage of work and just the stress, so using my, just thinking about myself as case material then, what does that mean for health workers as a whole. Is this what people do, they retreat into, you know, polarised identities? They're forced into it.'

A similar process was apparent with Roger. He was at pains to clarify that, when he said something critical about social work and social services, he meant social work management and not frontline social workers. He pointed out how much he had enjoyed his previous role with the Early Intervention Service (EIS) team before he transferred to Southville. At EIS he provided intensive support to young people experiencing psychosis, and he was able to meet each service user on his caseload three times a week. By contrast, at the CMHT, he was required to spend most of his time on the computer. Roger said he "liked the way it used to be. I do the nursing, Kerry [occupational therapist] does the work thing, you [social worker] do the social, not this generic thing". He then paused to reflect on this. He asked me if I was old enough to remember the introduction of the purchaser/provider split in social services. He then recounted an interaction with a long-serving social worker called Fred Fletcher back in the 1990s. Fred had described to Roger the damage the purchaser/provider split had done to social work, telling him: "I can't do this job anymore. My whole career, it's finished." After Roger told me that, he looked away. When he turned back, I saw frustration tinged with sadness on his face. "I've turned into Fred Fletcher," he said.

In both these examples, James and Roger shifted from their earlier analyses that were situated within a role actor frame and moved towards acknowledgement of themselves individually, but also of mental health workers more generally across occupational groups, in terms of their social class positioning. These reorientations highlight the potential to transcend the limitations of institutional 'role action' through horizontal solidarities and class-based collective agency. This does not mean that such solidarities will automatically or necessarily arise, but that these are nonetheless an emergent possibility.

While limited, there were some embryonic indicators of such developments. One example was an article informally circulated by email among social workers, nurses and the occupational therapist at Southville CMHT. It was forwarded to me by social worker Constance, who implored me to read it as team members discussed its contents enthusiastically in the office. The article was authored by an anonymous social worker[7] and written in an eloquent and bitingly satirical manner. It argued that the interdisciplinary power struggle, often characterised by tensions around social and medical models, is now submerged beneath a more important battle against a 'crude business ethic' in NHS mental health services. As a result, the power relations within the team between doctors and other practitioners are 'not as important as the power relations between clinical staff and management. For this reason, it is imperative we create an alliance of identities, a joint radical stance across the professions.'

An example of the potentials for that sort of alliance was the development of localised links between Roger and social worker Alan, who were UNISON trade union representatives for Southville's NHS and social work staff respectively. They worked together on a campaign against service cuts and increased workloads within the Trust. While this was initiated by social workers, Alan and Roger sought to mobilise staff from across occupational groups by developing a joint statement and petition.

Although not directly evoked in the article that was circulated, a further possibility for class-based forms of collective agency is that of cross-sectional service user–worker alliances to mobilise for services that are both better funded and more democratically organised (Sedgwick, 2015). Such orientations were evident in a small number of examples. These included a lobby outside the Middletown Centre mental health unit against Trust cuts and bed reductions, organised by local NHS campaigners and attended by service users, trade unionists, health and social workers and anti-austerity activists that took place during my fieldwork. Others were the coordination between Roger, UNISON activists and service user governors to intervene at Trust Board meetings, and staff support for service users around the closure of the Walk-In service. Faced with the twin challenges of managerial dominance and strenuous welfarism, such developments that seek to draw diverse occupational groups and service users together in political projects of collective agency are a reminder of the progressive impulse or 'radical kernel' contained within certain modes of welfare professionalism (Ferguson, 2009).

Also visible were forms of individual agency that challenged the limits of dominant injunctions for practitioners to orient primarily to the demands of informational work. In earlier chapters, practitioners described baulking at defensive practices of monitoring '"sleep, mood and meds" that were underpinned by neoliberal logics and the directional tendencies, such as biomedical residualism, to which they give rise. Consequently, there were multiple instances of workers striving to maintain social-relational and community-oriented forms of practice alongside service users in spite of these pressures. These micro-level forms of resistance were oriented to a countervailing tendency of ethico-political professionalism. This manifested as a defence of occupational autonomy and user-centred practice, and through direct and indirect challenges to punitive forms of managerialism.

This chapter has elaborated one particularly significant organisational effect of the neoliberalisation of the mental health system: the intensification of punitive managerial control and its harmful effects. This was enabled through institutional reforms, which included the marginalisation of collective mechanisms of trade union representation. These processes of organisational restructuring sought to impose a new informational order and marginalise older social-relational approaches and temporalities by means of an institutional culture of 'targets and terror', oriented to disciplining and punishing deviations from these licenced modalities. In response to these developments, practitioners, predominantly, oriented to institutional role action, which tended to reproduce these hierarchical environments and reinforce fragmentation and competition between occupational groups. However, there were some (more limited) examples of individual and collective agency to resist these dominant tendencies. In mobilising forms of solidarity with service users and across occupational groups while defending ethically oriented professional identities, such agential identifications embody an emergent potential to go beyond the reproduction of neoliberal service structures. This alternative offers hints of the possibilities for a progressive and democratic reshaping or even transforming of welfare structures and relations, and thereby of the forms of knowledge and practice articulated and enacted within them.

PART III

Theorising knowledge and practice

8

Temporality and situational logics in the labour process

In Part II, chapters 2-7, I explored the lived experiences of workers and service users at Southville Community Mental Health Team (CMHT) and then the Rehabilitation and Recovery Team (RRT). I briefly noted how situational logics and the strategic directional tendencies they generate shaped people's ideas and actions within this setting. In Part III, the next two chapters of the book, I will bring the concepts of situational logic, strategic directional tendency and the wider theoretical framework of Emergentist Marxism (EM) into closer focus. In the current chapter, I begin with a comprehensive overview of EM, including an account of political economy and the labour process as a basis for exploring the interplay of structure, culture and agency within mental health services. This provides a foundation from which the role of situational logics in shaping strategic directional tendencies in mental health services can be explained.

Before I begin this overview of EM, I will briefly outline the argument to be developed over the course of the chapter. I propose that the organisational landscape of public services is reshaped over time according to the needs of capital through processes of subsumption. However, due to the partial and uneven nature of subsumption, aspects of past conjunctural settlements remain embedded in the present in the form of multiple, sedimented material structures and ideational frameworks. Consequently, repurposed 'remnants' of older welfare settlements (such as biomedical models and custodialism) endure alongside newer emergent features (for example, informational practice systems and individual responsibilisation). As practitioners and service users navigate this uneven and differentiated terrain, the alignments and frictions between novel emergent and sedimented features create situational logics that play a crucial role in shaping and conditioning which types of practice and forms of knowledge are enacted and articulated. Within community mental health services, the dominant situational logic under neoliberalism generates 'strategic directional tendencies' towards *biomedical residualism* and *custodial paternalism*. However, these directional tendencies also engender resistance. Consequently, a 'countervailing directional tendency' towards *ethico-political professionalism* is also visible within this setting.

Political economy and levels of scale

EM is a theoretical framework that draws on, but significantly adapts, Archer's (1995) morphogenetic/morphostatic (M/M) model. It does so by developing a distinctive sociohistorical materialist account of agency and structure (Creaven, 2000, 2007), underpinned by critical realist meta-theory (Bhaskar, 1998). The latter is a philosophical ontology that specifies material reality as stratified (Creaven, 2000). The premise here is that the phenomena of the social world occur in open systems and thus their complex co-determination requires a conception of reality as comprised of multiple distinct mechanisms operating at a number of emergent and interacting levels (Bhaskar, 2010).[1]

I identify three levels of scale as particularly relevant for understanding the dynamics and effects of mental health service reform. These are the *macro* level of political economy shaping the particular form of the welfare state, for example, neoliberalism; the *meso* level, comprising occupational (that is, disciplinary/theoretical knowledge and professional roles, and interprofessional relations/division of labour) and organisational structures (for example, managerialism and the reconfiguration of occupational roles); and the *micro* level, that is, the contexts for interpersonal interactions and situated forms of knowledge (Pilgrim and Rogers, 1999; Hyde et al, 2016).

As this suggests, the historical reconfiguration of welfare regimes and consequent reconstitution of forms of professional knowledge and practice are the outcome of broader socioeconomic, political and ideational processes. More specifically, the political economy of the welfare state constitutes both the enabling condition for, and boundary limit on, policy-driven reconfigurations of meso-level organisational and occupational processes (Archer, 1995; Pilgrim, 2015). For EM, a central analytical concern is the interrelationship between the layers of the political economy and forms of agency within organisational labour processes. This is because, under capitalism, the labour process has a dual role, both fundamentally shaping and mediating the material needs and interests of people, while also providing the basis for capital accumulation (Creaven, 2000, 2007; Thompson and Vincent, 2010).

To examine this interface between macro-level political economy, meso-level organisational structures and the micro contingencies of practitioners' and service users' 'street-level' interpersonal interactions and conceptualisations, I draw on a labour process theory (LPT) approach within a wider EM framework (Thompson and Vincent, 2010).

The labour process

As noted in Chapter 1, neoliberal marketisation and New Public Management (NPM) have led to constraints on public sector professionals' control of their work practices, which are, increasingly, defined by employing organisations or the state (Evetts, 2010, 2011) within the context of market-oriented performance mechanisms (Harris, 2003). These changes in the material lived realities of work are linked to wider processes of capitalist restructuring. LPT begins from a conception of capitalism as a systemic whole, and the identification of labour's role in the creation of value within this (Braverman, 1974; Thompson and Vincent, 2010). The labour process under capitalism is regarded not only as a means to create use values (useful commodities) but also surplus value (profit) and thereby ensure the expansion and accumulation of capital.

While the labour process of public sector employees is not directly oriented to capital accumulation in the same way as those in the private sector, the welfare state is wholly integral to the functioning of capitalism.[2] Consequently, although workers in the public sector National Health Service (NHS) and social services do not (in the main) produce commodities directly,[3] their labour nonetheless adds to the amount of value produced collectively within the system as a whole. It thus creates indirect surplus value for capital (Umney, 2018).

Moreover, as producers of value, frontline public sector workers should be considered members of the working class and, although not (predominantly) productive of profit, such work remains subject to wider logics of accumulation within the capitalist economy (Reid, 2003). This broader environment of capitalism generates and imposes on the state particular political-economic imperatives and countervailing pressures. On the one hand, in so far as its provisions are the outcome of capital–labour struggles, the welfare state constitutes a 'social wage' while it also functions to maintain social cohesion (Ferguson et al, 2002). On the other hand, health and welfare provision reflects the needs of capital for social reproduction of the workforce (Bhattacharya, 2017), alongside demands on the state from its constituent capitals to reduce their costs in the form of corporate tax reductions (Carter and Stevenson, 2012).

Amid these tensions and ambiguities:

[S]tates come under the same pressure as do big capitals when faced with sudden competition – the pressure to restructure and reorganise their operations so as to accord with the law of value … this means trying to impose work measurement and payment schemes on welfare sector employees similar to those within the most competitive industrial firms. (Harman, 2010, p 138)

This highlights the way in which the demands of competition under capitalism have significant effects across the public as well as private sectors and reflects a broader imperative that underpins the labour process: to constantly renew production in order to increase labour productivity. This has implications for the composition of skills within, and structure of, the workforce (Hall, 2010), and may lead, for instance, to increases in the division of labour (Carter and Stevenson, 2012).

Alongside this, LPT identifies two other interrelated dynamics. These are the 'control imperative', or the need for management strategies to ensure maximisation of surplus value extracted from purchased labour power and, related to this, the 'structured antagonism' that characterises capital–labour relations in the workplace (Hall, 2010; Thompson and Vincent, 2010).

Strenuous welfarism

The discussion now turns to a more recent elaboration of LPT: 'strenuous welfarism' (Law and Mooney, 2007). This utilises and builds on the themes just described by identifying particular emergent trends in the reshaping of the labour process in public sector health and welfare work. Strenuous welfarism offers an effective means for understanding both transformations of work in neoliberalising mental health services and the temporal and affective pressures arising from these that were so prominent in the fieldwork chapters.

Chapter 1 noted that NHS and Community Care Act reforms in the 1990s led to significant changes in internal managerial cultures within NHS mental health services, with the adoption of 'quasi-business' and consumerist discourses modelled on the private sector. Consequently, practitioners' locus of technical control shifted during this period with the 'top-down' implementation of standardised procedures and performance audit regimes monitored by information and communication technologies (ICT), resulting in reduced discretion at the front line (Harris, 1998, 2003).

The implications of this were outlined in Chapter 2, where 'strenuous welfarism' was utilised to convey the effects of reductions in worker autonomy in the context of neoliberal reform and technological innovation within the public sector labour process. Prominent features of these reconfigurations include a tendency towards calculable quantification to enable comparative indicators of performance in a quasi-market setting, which results in the attempt by institutions 'to transform the tacit knowledge embedded in particular disciplines and organisational settings into the kind of codified knowledge that could be made subject to generic managerial measurements and controls' (Law and Mooney, 2007, p 43). In this way, ICT facilitates both the restructuring of work processes to increase output and the intensification of managerial surveillance and control. The intensification of the relationship between workers and ICT through these technological changes is thus integral to the neoliberalisation of work (Moore et al, 2018).

These neoliberal transformations of the labour process, initiated by the extension and deepening of performance indicator regimes and then further facilitated by ICT developments, have had multiple effects. These include increased administrative burdens that reduce time for the care and support of service users, the flexible intensification of worker effort and the loss of breathing space and porous time. This brings into focus the significant temporal implications of neoliberal labour process restructuring within this setting. Moreover, when workers align their practice with target-oriented demands in order to protect themselves from the potential for disciplinary interventions from senior managers, then the affective embodied and relational dimensions of worker–service user interaction are negatively impacted. However, such relational tensions and processes of disengagement are not captured by the mechanisms for measuring outputs via audits and targets.

Alongside these processes of work intensification, temporal reordering, affective demands and relational pressures, another development noted across the fieldwork chapters was the implementation of an increasingly complex division of labour. One prominent feature of this is workforce remodelling. This can be characterised by labour substitution, involving the transfer of less-skilled tasks from qualified professionals to lower-paid support workers (Carter and Stevenson, 2012). In mental health services this has taken the form of outsourcing to the voluntary sector, but also the creation of non-professional healthcare roles within the NHS, such as the assistant practitioner, employed on pay grades below those of newly qualified nurses (Henshall et al, 2018; Kessler and Spilsbury, 2019). Remodelling is also visible in processes of 'downbanding', or the reallocation of healthcare professionals to lower pay bands under the guise of workforce reprofiling, to reduce costs (Jones-Berry, 2016).

In relation to control imperatives, the growth of management hierarchies (or 'creeping managerialism') has been identified as a mechanism designed to further drive up output and productivity via measurement of key performance indicators (KPIs) (Carter et al, 2010). The organisational atmosphere of 'targets and terror' (Bevan and Hood, 2006) generated by these neoliberal transformation processes was highlighted in Chapters 6 and 7.

However, these processes unfold in complex, uneven and incomplete ways. Moreover, in the context of a highly stratified labour force, diverse groups of workers are affected differently. There is an inherent tension between processes of bureaucratisation and deskilling of welfare professionals and the performative discretion and task autonomy of models of professionalism (Harris, 2003; Law and Mooney, 2007). As a result: '[E]ven under strenuous welfare regimes, work typically retains something of the character of an artisanal labour process where some discretion is retained over how to carry out predetermined tasks' (Law and Mooney, 2007, p 45).

These 'discretionary spaces' provide opportunities to challenge the constraints imposed by neoliberal managerialism (Harris and White, 2009).

I discuss forms of agency oriented to resistance and recalcitrance briefly at the end of this chapter. However, first, I explore the causal tendencies in the labour process that underpin these uneven and differentiated organisational outcomes.

Subsumption, sedimentation and layered temporalities in the labour process

Organisational and labour process restructuring creates what Bhaskar (2008a, p 130) calls 'rhythmically differentially sedimented structures'. This describes the uneven spatial and temporal effects of processes of institutional reform, where aspects of the past remain embedded in the present. This was visible at Southville, for instance, in the co-existence, alongside 21st-century informational data management, of the artisanal aspects of post-war therapeutic relational approaches and 'archaic' custodial interventions reflecting the legacy of the asylum. The different temporal rhythms associated with each of these practices were noted in Chapter 3.

The processes through which such uneven and differentiated spatiotemporalities are generated have recently been explored in the work of Tomba (2013) and Harootunian (2015). These scholars have argued that they are caused by ongoing but also conflictual and incomplete processes of what Marx describes as 'subsumption'. This is the mechanism whereby labour shaped by non-capitalist social relations is integrated or subsumed into a labour process shaped by capital. In historical terms, subsumption in the 18th century initially involved only indirect control over labour processes by capital. Capitalists provided workers with tools and raw materials but traditional artisanal methods of production were maintained. This is known as formal subsumption. However, subsequently, capitalists assumed more direct control over production through transformations of the labour process via larger-scale modes of industrial manufacture involving more complex divisions of labour. This is referred to as real subsumption (Marx, 1990).[4] These processes of formal and real subsumption continue in contemporary capitalism, with ongoing incremental organisational and technological transformations of the labour process designed to realise increased productivity and commodification (Marx, 1990; Joyce, 2020). In this study, the notion of subsumption offers a crucial explanatory framework for the ongoing loss by mental health workers of the remaining elements of independence, discretion and control within the labour process and work tasks.

The subsumption of labour processes under capitalism generates a tendency towards synchronisation. This is because, in the encounter between capital and existing ways of working, the relative productive powers of older and newer labour processes are measured against each other using the yardstick of 'socially necessary labour-time'. The latter refers to the amount of time taken by a typical worker with average skill levels within a society to produce a commodity. This measure, by which value is assigned to the commodity to facilitate and regulate its exchange in markets, enables comparison between producers (Marx, 1990). Synchronisation takes place because temporal gaps between older and newer labour processes are highlighted by this medium of socially necessary labour-time in the context of increasingly integrated (national and global) markets (Tomba, 2013). The value of commodities produced through older, less efficient labour processes are higher and thus less competitive, so there is a pressure to discard practices, concepts and organisational forms associated with earlier phases of development and replace them with newer, more productive processes. Socially necessary labour-time thus functions as a 'universal chronometer' (Tomba, 2013, p.149), with processes of subsumption synchronising diverse labour processes through the imposition of a dominant temporality, and thereby reshaping the institutional environments of workplace and society.

These processes do not, however, produce homogeneity in the social and cultural structures on which they act, but the resultant effects are instead partial and uneven. This is because, while capital may comprehensively subsume and restructure some of the existing organisational forms it encounters, in other cases the situational demands, barriers or resistance encountered generate adaptations rather than transformations. Consequently, there are limits to synchronisation. While some practices, concepts and organisational forms associated with earlier institutional environments are discarded and replaced by newer structures, the residues (Harootunian, 2015), sediments or 'still unconquered remnants' (Marx, 1993, p 105) of other longstanding practices and ideas may be appropriated and repurposed to meet contemporary requirements.

Because public sector workers create indirect (and sometimes direct) surplus value for capital, these dynamics of subsumption and synchronisation are as applicable to labour processes in health and social care as they are to work in general under capitalism (Law and Mooney, 2007). Thus, subsumption and its countervailing tendencies produce tensions between homogeneity (due to synchronisation) and unevenness (the repurposing of 'sediments' of earlier systems) within the welfare state just as they do in the wider economy. These incomplete and partial processes reflect capital's adaptations to diverse political and economic demands but are also an outcome of the forms of resistance the system encounters. Consequently, a complex patchwork of transformations and sedimentations is produced within the 'ecological niche' (Hacking, 2002) of the welfare state. Although each new conjunctural settlement of the mental health system generates novel forms of institution and practice, existing welfare practices and ideologies are not fully displaced and significant traces of earlier forms of thought and action endure. These sedimented elements remain embedded within present practice modalities as both 'archaic remnants' and unrealised progressive potentialities on which current actors may draw (Harootunian, 2015).

In neoliberal mental health services, real subsumption is apparent in the way that labour processes based on older forms of relational-therapeutic practice are increasingly being reconfigured to foreground informational data production for health and social care markets and quasi-markets. However, these subsumption processes are uneven. Aspects of the 'archaic sediments' of custodial institutionalisation and the medically dominated hospital system continue to meet some contemporary demands of the capitalist state for forms of risk management within the ecosystem of neoliberal services, and so have been adapted and repurposed for this context. Moreover, many practitioners continue to identify with social-relational (therapeutic) approaches despite the pressures imposed by an informational labour process, so this feature also endures in the present. As a result of these multiple co-existing 'layers', mental health services are like a 'pentimento'[5] (Rhodes, 1993), with 'an ensemble of practices in their different temporalities, struggling to assert their primacy' (Thomas, 2009, p 284).

As this suggests, the unevenness generated by processes of subsumption and sedimentation have temporal implications. Practitioners and service users navigating this layered action environment encounter organisational structures characterised by a 'heterogeneous mix' of institutional, disciplinary and experiential temporalities (Harootunian, 2015, p 206). For example, long-term care coordination involves extended engagements between practitioners and service users consisting of a slower rhythm and an extended relational temporal horizon (*social-relational time*). This contrasts with duty work, which is characterised by brief and highly episodic interactions over the short term, underpinned by an accelerated task-focused and assessment-oriented rhythmic (*informational time*). Frictions emerge as the established social-relational disciplinary temporalities of professions such as social work and nursing, oriented to long-term casework, collide with new neoliberal managerialist temporalities based on short-term informational practices.

Practitioners and service users respond to the frictions, collisions and 'rhythmical contradictions' between divergent temporal orders, and the experiences of *temporal dissonance* associated with them, in multiple ways. These processes may cause stress and burnout (Rosa, 2017). But workers and service users also enact various forms of 'temporal agency' (Flaherty, 2011) in response to them. They may engage in a process of 'agentic synchronisation' between these different temporal layers, by 'synchroniz[ing] sometimes radically different temporalities entailing different durations, paces, frequencies, sequences and timings' (Vostal et al, 2019, p 799). However, such experiences may compel a second agentic response, that of resistance (Bensaïd, 2002). Temporal agency from below represents an important countervailing tendency to the 'top-down' synchronisation associated with subsumption processes. Tomba (2013, p 169) refers to this as the 'counter-times' of labour and social struggles.

The forms of recalcitrance and resistance that are engendered by points of structural antagonism and temporal contradiction within these organisational processes may be channelled through trade union structures or emerge in other more spontaneous forms (Ackroyd, and Thompson, 1999; Fairbrother and Poynter, 2001). In Chapter 7, Roger described forms of collective trade union activism, while in Chapters 2, 6 and elsewhere an ethico-political orientation among some practitioners was illustrated through small-scale 'quiet challenges' to managerialism in everyday practice (Harris and White, 2009). These included efforts to preserve relational and therapeutic spaces in the face of managerialist constraints and cuts, for instance the temporal agency demonstrated by Kath and Leslie in 'slowing down' clinic interactions or imperatives to discharge users. Another example is the exercise of professional discretion by Yvonne and Farooq in relation to assessments or community treatment orders (CTOs) to strategically circumvent organisational obstacles and thereby secure greater resources or liberties for service users. Preserving notions of professionalism through adherence to disciplinary temporalities (for example, Yvonne and Kath's efforts to maintain relationship-based practices) represented a countervailing tendency in opposition to the informational time constraints of neoliberal managerialism (Evetts, 2003). Many of these practices suggest a defence of ethical professionalism linked to values of social justice (Lavalette, 2007), a theme I return to later in this chapter, then explore in more detail in the next.

Structure, culture, agency and situational logics

As we have seen, the transformation of mental health services and their labour processes through subsumption has been uneven and incomplete, producing forms of institutional sedimentation. I now turn to the implications of these sedimented action environments for knowledge and practice in this setting. To examine this, I begin with EM's account of structure, culture and agency, and then situational logics. I argue that these logics, and the 'directional tendencies' within practice that they generate, play a significant role in shaping the ways that lived experiences of mental distress are understood and responded to in this context.

Structure and culture in EM

EM regards agency, structure and culture as ontologically distinct and mutually irreducible strata of reality, each with their own particular properties and powers. This stance thereby enables examination of the relationship and interplay between them. Moreover, by recognising that interactants always confront pre-existing structural and cultural forms that enable or constrain their activities, a temporal dimension is introduced. Structure and culture pre-date action, which human activity then reproduces (morphostasis) or occasionally transforms (morphogenesis). In this sense, structures and cultural forms shape or condition but do not determine agency. As noted earlier, EM foregrounds the structural dimensions of the labour process and associated forms of activity and contestation while retaining a non-reductive ontological orientation (Creaven, 2000).

While structure and culture are both emergent properties and have many parallel features, they are, nonetheless, different in kind. Structure refers to the relatively enduring material and relational 'parts' of a social system, for instance entities such as NHS community mental health services characterised by specific organisational relations between people, roles and material artefacts such as buildings. However, these structures are sedimented, so forms of 'archaic' hospital and custodial institutional arrangements and longer-established multiprofessional team models co-exist alongside a contemporary informational infrastructure, service-line management (SLM) and emerging active welfare-oriented occupational roles such as employment support worker.

Meanwhile, culture refers 'to the ensemble of ideological and ideational structures of a society (that is, systems of communication, meaning, legitimation and knowledge)' (Creaven, 2007, p 162). As with structures, there is sedimentation of cultural/ideational features in mental health services. Consequently, emergent ideational frameworks such as recovery exist alongside more longstanding bodies of knowledge[6] such as the biomedical model. Moreover, while formal theoretical knowledge (for example, models of mental distress) and applied forms of knowledge (such as professional ethical codes, local assessment protocols and so on) are human activity dependent, such discourses have causal powers in their own right once emergent from this activity (Archer, 1995). These forms of knowledge are, in this respect, 'objective'. They become sedimented within settings such as CMHTs as cultural forms that are encountered by future agents, although not in the sense of being a static, unchanging monolith. Rather, in so far as their externality in the public domain and relative autonomy from particular knowing subjects render them amenable to forms of agentic reflexivity and intervention, such sets of ideas may themselves be transformed as well as reproduced.[7] The ideational sediment of past activities in the form of the various models of mental distress thereby constitutes a material force, shaping but also itself conditioned and reshaped by human agency (Layder, 1997).[8]

Agency in EM

Together, structure and culture form 'a pre-existent "action-environment" of both material and cultural distributions, which agents inhabit and have to come to terms with in thought and deed' (Creaven, 2007, p 148). Therefore, as people encounter these differentially sedimented cultures (including bodies of knowledge) and structures (for example, entities such as mental health teams composed of organisational and occupational roles and relations), these structures/cultures shape their activities. However, the causal powers of people are independent and irreducible and so human action is not wholly determined by these structural and cultural forms. Instead, the causal powers of structures and cultures are mediated through social activity (Bhaskar, 1998).[9] Moreover, the nature of such activity is shaped by people's identities, which are multiply determined. This highlights EM's stratified conception of personal and social identity which, as Chapter 7 noted, specifies three interacting dimensions of embodied subject, role actor (in institutions) and agent (in society).

These identities are, furthermore, shaped and mediated by the (unequal) distributions of allocative and authoritative resources in society and the associated hierarchical social relations in which people find themselves involuntarily situated. For EM, structures of class inequality are of particular salience, though gendered, racialised and other forms of social stratification are also integral to this form of analysis. From these structured inequalities derive positional interests that motivate forms of social interaction, including social struggles.[10] While positional interests are objective, people's responses to them are not automatic but instead reflexively determined. However, in the context of relative scarcity of resources, opportunity costs are incurred by interactants who choose not to act in accordance with them. The way people respond to their situated conditions within a particular social or organisational environment, either individually (primary agency) or collectively utilising structural capacities that derive from the stratified socioeconomic and sociocultural environments in which they are enmeshed (collective agency),[11] determines whether society is reproduced, elaborated or transformed over time.[12]

Situational logics and directional tendencies in EM

The previous section has highlighted how the social structures and relations within which individuals find themselves involuntarily located define their objective positional interests and attendant opportunity costs, and offer them ideational resources through which to make sense of their situations. Structural and cultural influences thus operate by 'shaping the situations in which people find themselves [...] which are mediatory because they condition (without determining) different courses of action for those differently placed, by supplying different reasons to them' (Archer, 1995, p 201). It is the properties of these structural and cultural systems, including the contradictions and complementarities between them, that generate these objective influences or 'situational logics'. These logics shape people's daily experiences, and their scope and motivations for forms of action within particular institutional settings. They do not determine activity, however, because people retain an irreducible intentional capacity to 'choose between reasons', which acts as a mediator of these structural and cultural influences. Nonetheless, this introduces a directional tendency, with situational logics providing interactants with 'strategic directional guidance' in the form of encouragement towards, or discouragement from, certain courses of action (Creaven, 2000).

An important implication of this for the analysis of situational logics in complex institutional settings is that particular structural and cultural phenomena do not operate as a form of hydraulic socialisation with a propensity to directly determine how agents think and act. In other words, there is not one structural or cultural emergent feature that 'hydraulically' determines and homogenises ideas and practices. For while each structural and cultural form considered in isolation (known as a 'first-order emergent' in EM) exerts its own causal effects, organisational settings such as healthcare systems are composed of multiple interacting structural and cultural elements. Moreover, these may be in a more or less mutually conflictual or complementary relation with each other. The outcomes of the interactions between two or more of these first-order mechanisms produce their own distinctive causal properties and powers, which are called 'second-order emergents'. These second-order features, and the positional and ideational conflicts or compatibilities integral to them, shape people's reflexive evaluations of their circumstances both by furnishing agents with material (interest-based) and normative 'reasons for action' and by highlighting opportunity costs to be avoided. In this way, second-order emergents define the situational logics experienced by people in institutional settings, and create 'directional tendencies' for action in the form of contradictions which constrain activities or alignments which enable them (Creaven, 2000).

Situational logics and directional tendencies in mental health services

The previous section has noted the importance of differentiating first-order and second-order emergent properties in order to analyse their interrelationships. This, it is argued, provides a critical basis for understanding the interactions between structural, cultural and agential processes that shape the articulation of ideas and practices within complex organisational action-environments such as mental health services. This enables a move beyond forms of theoretical reductionism that foreground the 'hydraulic' and homogenising determination of ideas and practices through a single, dominant structural or cultural emergent feature. This kind of reductionism is visible, for instance, in the work of Burstow (2015)[13], where mental health services are constructed as dominated by a monolithic biomedical-psychiatric hegemon. However, for EM, such a state of affairs is untenable within complex environments such as CMHTs and RRTs, where a multiplicity of material structures and ideational frameworks emerge and endure, co-exist and are contested. This is because, while each 'first-order emergent' structure in mental health services (such as informational practice systems or medically-dominated hierarchies) or cultural form (for example biomedical models and critical ethico-political orientations) exerts its own causal effects, these multiple structural and cultural phenomena have a tendency to coalesce into mutual alignments or frictions within this ecological niche. It is the second-order emergents which arise through this process, and the directional tendencies they generate, that play a critical role in shaping the concepts and activities in use within this organisational system.

Having established the utility of delineating first-order and second-order emergent properties, I will now outline the first-order emergent features that remain sedimented and thus salient within the current conjunctural settlement of neoliberal mental health services, and highlight their combination into second-order emergents that shape situational logics in this context. I then describe three 'directional tendencies' associated with these situational logics and their conditioning influence on ideas and practices within this institutional setting.

As noted in Chapter 1, the current neoliberal iteration of services is characterised by two novel (first-order) emergent features. The first is an *informational practice system*, which has arisen to meet the requirements of the dominant market-oriented and risk-management policy frameworks that now structure work routines. These new organisational arrangements involve a redesigned labour process, reoriented towards the processing of digital data required for KPIs, care plans, assessments, risk assessments and so on. This has also involved the creation of new service pathways for service users, temporally and spatially redesigned to reflect the new priorities centred on performance metrics and risk actuarialism. While the *informational practice system* is oriented to production processes for healthcare markets, the second emergent feature, *individual responsibilisation*, is a normative and ideational intervention seeking to reshape consumption practices by service users. This value orientation underpins measures such as personal budgets and personalisation, and practices including psychoeducation and self-care strategies. These all seek to embed parsimonious resource utilisation through self-management and short-term modes of provision.

Beyond the contemporary neoliberal layer, two emergent features of the post-war community care settlement remain visible within this setting. The most significant of these are the various forms of *social-relational approach*. These include modalities of therapy and counselling interventions (which also continue to influence practices within casework and care coordination), but also community work approaches. A second, less prominent but nonetheless visible feature is an *ethico-political orientation*. This refers to politico-normative theories and forms of praxis drawing on radical traditions such as critical and liberatory theory, service user/survivor movements, critical iterations of service user involvement, antipsychiatry and antidiscriminatory perspectives. Although, admittedly, these exist at the margins of mainstream services, their influence on activities within this setting can nonetheless be detected.

The next emergent feature, the *biomedical model*, rose to full prominence both as a nosology and set of practices during the early 20th century, when it became an integral element and enabler of the development of the hospital system. However this framework, and associated practices including diagnosis, biomedical aetiological theories, and treatment and monitoring via psychotropic medication (a manifestation of pharmaceuticalisation), remains extremely prominent within the contemporary context. Closely related to this is the other enduring emergent feature that arose during this earlier settlement, the consolidation of *medical dominance* through the displacement of judicial powers that established psychiatry at the apex of a hospital-based professional hierarchy. This feature underpins a paternalist orientation towards patients/service users that endures into the present.

The final two sedimented emergent features are a legacy of the conjunctural settlement of the 19th-century asylum, which developed as a means to impose forms of segregative control on populations constructed as 'deviant' and a threat to the developing industrial capitalist order (Scull, 1977). The first, *custodialism*, endures as a restrictive form of institutionalised organisational practice. The second emergent feature, the *discourse of danger and violence* associated with mental distress, relates closely to the first, and operates to provide justification for such custodial interventions. Table 8.1 lists the conjunctural settlements and their corresponding first-order emergent features.

Having set out the various first-order emergent features that remain prominent within neoliberal mental health services, the chapter now turns to the situational logics that emerge at the second-order interactional nexus between these multiple first-order mechanisms. In order to elaborate these, it is necessary to illustrate the kinds of circumstances under which such logics and their associated directional tendencies become more visible.

Table 8.1: First-order emergent features

Conjunctural settlement	First-order emergent features
Neoliberal	Informational practice system (oriented to markets and risk)
	Individual responsibilisation
Community care	Social-relational approaches
	Ethico-political orientation
Biomedical hospital	Medical dominance
	Biomedical model
Asylum	Custodialism
	Discourse of danger and violence

Practitioner and service responses to users' transitions between the status of 'stable' and that of 'acute' (or 'relapse', 'in crisis'), detailed earlier in the study, often vividly revealed prominent institutional pressures, or situational logics, shaped by differential distributions of power and resources. Within neoliberal mental health services, these took the form of top-down sociopolitical and organisational demands to contain costs and manage risk. These institutional constraints came more clearly into focus at these points of transition or 'crisis' for service users, and shaped the conditions of possibility for practice in determinate ways. Under these conditions, alignments and complementarities between certain models of mental distress and modes of practice tended to be more effective in realising such organisational demands. These contextual pressures thus narrowed practitioners' scope for action by generating strategic directional tendencies towards certain ways of thinking and acting within this setting, most prominently 'biomedical residualism', and 'custodial paternalism'.

However, while dominant situational logics shape and condition activity within this setting, because of human reflexivity they do not determine it. People sometimes chose to act against their vested interests within this organisational context, and instead align with their preferred values-based and political positions. Consequently, a countervailing directional tendency from below, 'ethico-political professionalism', was also visible. This was in a relationship of mutual tension to top-down situational logics insofar as it reflected a set of institutional and ethico-political dynamics that challenged dominant orientations towards market efficiencies and defensive risk management. Thus, the tensions and shifts by practitioners between models and modes of practice that were discernible at these transition or 'crisis' points for service users reflected both alignments with but also resistance to dominant 'directional tendencies'. These tendencies, and the second-order emergents underpinning them, will now be described in more detail.

Table 8.2: Strategic directional tendency of biomedical residualism

First-order emergent features	Strategic directional tendency (generated by situational logic)
Informational practice system	**Biomedical residualism**
Individual responsibilisation	
Biomedical model	
Discourse of danger and violence	

The first strategic directional tendency, characterised as *biomedical residualism* (see Table 8.2), was prominent in neoliberal services during service users' 'stable phase'. The changes in the ways that practitioners and service users interacted that were generated by this tendency were presented in Chapter 2. Indicators of this tendency include terms such as "hit and run" used by community mental health nurse (CMHN) Kath to disparagingly describe the time constraints that resulted in increasingly brief meetings with service users, and the defensive focus on checking users' "sleep, mood and meds" noted by Evelyn.

As this suggests, practitioners' aspirations to mobilise their preferred therapeutic (social-relational) modalities in work with service users was increasingly constrained by certain emergent features of the CMHT and later RRT. These included the *informational practice system*, introduced as a result of neoliberal reform, which limited practitioners' time for relationship-based approaches. These constraints on relational support were, in turn, legitimised by the promulgation of *individual responsibilisation*, which manifests as a moral injunction for service users to self-manage in the context of cuts. Alongside this, the re-emergence of older *discourses of danger and violence* associated with madness and mental distress has foregrounded an emphasis on risk management at a moment when practitioners' temporal capacities to do so through relationships have become more limited. In this context, another longstanding feature, the *biomedical model*, offered an alternative (defensive) means to manage risk via medication compliance.

Thus, these four relatively complementary first-order emergent features aligned to generate a distinctive situational logic, which created a directional tendency towards *biomedical residualism* in the particular 'ecological niche' created by the neoliberalisation of mental health services. This strategic directional tendency limited practitioners' interactions with service users to brief interventions focused on monitoring medication, and thereby marginalised social-relational approaches. However, this 'real determinate absence' (Creaven, 2002, p 85) of social approaches had its own causal implications in terms of engendering resistance (this will be discussed below in relation to the third countervailing tendency).

Table 8.3: Strategic directional tendency of custodial paternalism

First-order emergent features	Strategic directional tendency (generated by situational logic)
Biomedical model	Custodial paternalism
Medical dominance	
Discourse of danger and violence	
Custodialism	

The second strategic directional tendency, *custodial paternalism* (see Table 8.3), is closely related to the first. This tendency was prominent in neoliberal services during service users' 'crisis phase'. This was often visible where users were perceived not to have complied with or posed challenges to residualising and responsibilising tendencies within services, representing a punitive response within the lacunae of neoliberal psychocentric injunctions. This second constellation of ideas and practices was emergent from the prominent negative risk-oriented elements of mental health policy. It combined the repurposed 'archaic' sedimented features of *custodialism* and *discourses of danger* from the asylum era, and the *biomedical model* and *medical dominance* associated with the hospital system. It manifested organisationally as biomedically focused precautionary prudentialism[14] in the form of CTOs, re-institutionalisation and expanding forensic provision (Hare Duke et al, 2018). This foregrounds the way that situational logics under neoliberalism embed a strategic directional tendency or institutional path (Maielli, 2015) characterised by defensive risk management, with coercive and restrictive interventions utilised as a means to enforce biomedical treatment compliance and segregate purportedly risky populations (Pilgrim, 2015).

An exemplar of custodial paternalism was the response to the incident involving Manu at the hostel described in Chapter 4. CMHN Abbie focused on what she regarded as Manu's difficulty in taking responsibility for his behaviour, legitimising a care plan involving treatment within forensic services to resolve the risk-related barriers to placement that she was experiencing. Abbie's situational interpretation thus appeared to be shaped by the wider organisational exigencies associated with this situational logic. With reference to the same situation, James acknowledged that the initial focus of the care plan, combining what he described as institutionalisation, therapy and biomedical treatment, did not produce a successful outcome. James considered this to be a consequence of the custodial aspect of the strategy creating forms of dependency that undermined the therapeutic goal – for Manu to develop independent living skills. James's concern can be reconstructed as a contradiction between custodial paternalism (the alignment of custodialism, risk management and biomedical treatment) and

Table 8.4: Countervailing directional tendency of ethico-political professionalism

First-order emergent features	Countervailing directional tendency (generated by situational logic)
Social-relational approaches	**Ethico-political professionalism**
Ethico-political orientation	

the community placement (social-relational approach). Frictions emerged because the social-relational placement intervention was incompatible with the wider situational logic. This dominant logic ultimately imposed a strategic directional tendency towards an outcome of forensic intervention in spite of James's intentions and preferred modes of practice.

However, sometimes practitioners and service users resisted dominant logics and their associated directional tendencies. This is illustrated by a third countervailing tendency of *ethico-political professionalism* (see Table 8.4). This was visible within neoliberal services during service users' 'stable phase', although is significantly less prominent than biomedical residualism. The reason for these differentiated levels of visibility is that, while biomedical residualism is enabled by complementarities between a number of contemporary emergent features of mental health services, the social-relational and critical/radical approaches that combine to generate the countervailing directional tendency of ethico-political professionalism are in tension with currently dominant situational logics under neoliberalism.

Nonetheless, there were numerous examples of practitioners seeking to enact relational and participatory practices that reflected deeper rather than surface-level engagements with service users. These were outlined in Chapter 2 and elsewhere. These practices were powered by democratic ethico-political commitments. The stratified understanding of action in EM offers analytic purchase on how positional interests shape these kinds of ethico-political challenges to dominant logics and directional tendencies under neoliberalism through individual or collective forms of agency oriented to contesting prevailing ideas, practices, power relations and resources. The interface in EM between social agency and institutional role action sheds further light on this, and its implications for forms of recalcitrance and resistance will be discussed in greater detail in the next chapter.

In summary, my argument here is that the dominant situational logic under neoliberalism generates strategic directional tendencies within community mental health services towards *biomedical residualism* and *custodial paternalism*. However, these directional tendencies also engender resistance. Consequently, a countervailing directional tendency towards *ethico-political professionalism* is also visible within this setting. My claim is not that these situational logics and directional tendencies are exhaustive of those that are discernible in this setting. Rather, they are illustrative of currently prominent tendencies.

As the six fieldwork chapters have shown, these dominant logics and associated directional tendencies illustrate how institutional dynamics have eroded spaces for discretionary responses by practitioners to service users' needs. During the 'stable phase' of work with service users, such tendencies manifested as the closing down of spaces for social-relational support. During the 'crisis phase', these tendencies were visible in the foregrounding of coercive and custodial interventions and the limited spaces for alternatives to these. The situational logics that arise under neoliberalism, and the directional tendencies associated with them, thus have significant implications for the kinds of knowledges and practices that can be articulated and enacted in this context.

It is in this latter regard, I argue, that the strengths of an EM orientation are most apparent. This approach recognises and highlights the importance and centrality of the shift from social-relational approaches under community care to a dominant informational orientation in the neoliberal era. However, its analytical value is in also going beyond this to account for the enduring presence of features such as the biomedical model and custodialism (as well as social-relational practices), despite these dominant informational tendencies. It does so by offering a comprehensive explanatory framework theorising subsumption and sedimentation processes within mental health services, their role in creating an uneven, differentiated and layered terrain, and the way the latter shapes articulations of knowledge and practice. Subsumption is identified as important because it generates the dominant processes of informational reconfiguration under neoliberalism. But sedimentation too has significant effects. The increasingly residualised and restrictive dynamics of services under neoliberal austerity represent an ecological niche with which the 'archaic sediments' of biomedical and custodial interventions have proven highly compatible.

However, these restrictive practices and the temporal constraints associated with them generate dissonances and engender resistance among some practitioners and service users. This, in turn, reveals a third element, the politico-normative impulses that drive the mobilisation of social-relational approaches (another 'archaic remnant', but one that reflects resistance to dominant trends in provision) as well as ethico-political practices (influenced by the yet-to-be fully realised progressive potentialities of liberatory movements and radical models of practice). The EM approach enables an understanding of these complex and competing dynamics through its account of mental health services as a layered domain where practitioners and service users encounter newly emergent and sedimented structural and cultural features that co-exist in both complementary and conflictual relationships. Moreover, the EM framework also crucially highlights that it is through the activities and interactions of practitioners, service users and others that forms of knowledge, practice and wider mental health systems themselves tend to be reproduced but may also, potentially, be transformed.

The implications of these critical and transformative forms of agency for dominant logics and directional tendencies and, in particular, for countervailing ethico-political trends will be examined in the next chapter.

9

Biomedical residualism and
its discontents

This chapter begins by exploring discontent with currently dominant situational logics and associated directional tendencies, before identifying countervailing logics, tendencies and forms of resistance. It then goes on to consider how the latter might inform the development of alternative 'thick' social-relational approaches within mental health services, and the collective agents and particular forms of agency through which these might be realised.

Discontent with biomedical residualism (and custodial paternalism)

The previous chapter provided a detailed account of the dominant logics, and strategic directional tendencies of biomedical residualism and custodial paternalism generated by them, that have emerged in the context of neoliberalising mental health services. While there were a range of responses to these developments, the fieldwork chapters illustrated that critical perspectives were widespread among practitioners and service users. A common theme animating this 'discontent' was that valued opportunities for social and relational forms of support were increasingly limited within this setting. Instead, biomedical and residualised forms of practice were predominant. However, as Chapter 1 noted, there has been a nominal shift in mental health policy from a predominantly biomedical orientation towards a more recovery-focused social inclusion agenda in recent years. Thus, at the ideational level these policy positions might appear to suggest a more favourable terrain for social and relational perspectives for understanding and responding to mental distress. This first section of the chapter will build on the analysis developed across the previous chapters to demonstrate how emergent structural conditions during the neoliberal era have constituted a barrier to such developments.

Situational logics and disciplining mechanisms

In the previous chapter I focused primarily on the 'top-down' situational logics and the directional tendencies associated with processes of neoliberalisation. These powerful logics and tendencies shaped practitioner activities in ways that reproduced residualised and biomedically oriented forms of intervention. Sometimes this was because logics generated 'strategic directional guidance' that influenced practitioners' rationalisations or situational interpretations in ways that encouraged alignments with these tendencies. More frequently, however, when reflecting on these dynamics, practitioners stressed a lack of identification with these modes of practice. Rather, in many instances, the logic operated through the imposition of opportunity costs on practitioners who defied dominant logics by not acting in accordance with them.

These opportunity costs became visible through the penalties experienced by those who chose or were forced to pay them. These ranged from the temporal costs of working extra hours during the evenings to accommodate the additional time commitments of relational casework (for example, Yvonne and Kath), or the stresses generated by conflicts with managers over 'green dashboard' targets (for example, Leslie). Perhaps most striking are the career and reputational penalties that arose from Evelyn's subjection to disciplinary procedures and exit from the Trust following her perceived failures to adhere to top-down informational demands in a defensive 'inquiry culture'. Although not comparable to the levels of social harm experienced by many service users facing the deeply damaging impacts of austerity cuts through 'discharge deaths' and 'benefits distress' (Moth and Lavalette, 2017; Beresford, 2019; Moth, forthcoming b), such penalties nonetheless exerted a significant toll on practitioners. Moreover, the widespread fear (and sometimes actuality) of these negative consequences functioned as a powerful disciplining mechanism, creating significant pressures towards adherence to dominant logics.

Countervailing logics, directional tendencies and resistance

Nonetheless, there were numerous examples of practitioners identifying sufficiently with countervailing (for example, ethical or political) motivations to reject or resist these pressures. In this section, I identify and examine the countervailing logics and tendencies from below that informed these stances as actors and agents sought to circumvent, implement alternatives to or directly resist these situational logics from above. This discussion will be developed in two sections, the first describing forms of social-relational practice in the interstices of dominant logics under neoliberalism, the second elucidating interventions that represented a more direct challenge to informational orientations and associated tendencies towards biomedical residualism. These countervailing directional tendencies are theorised as 'ethico-political professionalism'.

Preserving social-relational spaces

Strenuous welfarism led to temporal constraints during the Community Mental Health Team (CMHT) phase of the neoliberal era, and thus practices associated with the strategic directional tendency of biomedical residualism were widely visible. Nonetheless, at times, practitioners utilised remaining pockets of porous time to maintain social-relational spaces for forms of preventive or therapeutic casework, including in-depth relationship-based practice, collective forms of groupwork and community work. Examples include Evelyn's work with Harriet on medication reduction and Leslie's life story work with Ray utilising the 'tree of life' tool. Another example is the development of relational initiatives such as the 'My Story' narrative workshops. Leslie explained that these had replaced a series of sessions providing psychoeducation (that is, providing information for service users/carers on psychiatric diagnosis/prognosis/treatment) run by the Trust. The workshops thus heralded an important ideational shift from an individual-biomedical to a social-relational approach. The methodology also changed from a didactic to a participatory orientation with the promotion of service user involvement and expertise visible in Harriet's role as workshop co-organiser and co-facilitator alongside Evelyn and Leslie. This participatory and egalitarian ethos was apparent in the avoidance of overt demarcation of service user and practitioner participants within sessions, and participants repositioned from passive consumers of information to actively engaged in narrative practices during the workshops. My Story workshops also sought to create spaces accessible to wider communities, thus challenging the restrictions of eligibility criteria and going beyond dominant individualised forms of practice within services.

This wider-scale approach is also visible in the community work orientation of social worker Farooq. He strongly advocated the need for the service to develop greater cultural sensitivity and awareness in supporting members of the British Pakistani community resident in the local area. Since joining the CMHT, Farooq had sought to actively engage in such practices as far as possible, including involvement in conducting research and publishing a report for the Trust on community needs and engagement. However, he expressed concern about the lack of ongoing support for implementing the findings of the report among senior management within the Trust and added that the individualised nature of practice models also constituted a barrier to such community work approaches.

However, the intensification of strenuous welfarism that accompanied the service-line management (SLM) reconfiguration and implementation of the Rehabilitation and Recovery Team (RRT) model led to further limitations on porous time. This resulted in challenges for practitioners in maintaining relational casework spaces with service users, and consequently some sought to insert some relational work into informational and managerial spaces. An example was Kath's depot clinic where, in apparently inhospitable conditions, she sought to carve out spaces for relationality that challenged the dominant institutional temporality. Thus, instead of creating/maintaining autonomous relational spaces in the interstices between informational demands, practitioners were increasingly forced to try to carve out relational moments within the informational spaces themselves.

These interstitial forms of social-relational practice represent a continuity with dominant practice modalities during the community care era. However, while these approaches would have been regarded as mainstream during that conjunctural settlement, they have become increasingly inconsistent with contemporary biomedical residualist logics and associated informational practice under neoliberalism. Consequently, while these relational modalities are not radical in themselves, engaging in such practices involved practitioners challenging currently prevailing logics and directional tendencies in practice.

Countervailing directional tendencies of ethico-political professionalism

As well as holding on to these relational interventions, there was also evidence of more direct contestation of dominant situational logics and strategic directional tendencies. These often drew on conceptions of professional values as a countervailing mechanism of challenge and resistance to New Public Management (NPM) reforms (Ackroyd et al, 2007; Lavalette, 2007). As noted in the last chapter, these politico-normative commitments prompted practitioners to engage in forms of recalcitrant activity that brought together an *ethico-political orientation* and *social-relational approaches* to generate a countervailing tendency of *ethico-political professionalism*. This logic was driven by the politico-normative commitments of some practitioners to 'absent the relational absences' of biomedical residualism (Creaven, 2002; Bhaskar, 2008a).

There were numerous examples of micro-level forms of resistance to organisational demands. The RRT saw intensified pressure on practitioners for increased throughput by discharging care-coordinated service users who were not perceived to have current high levels of need and risk. However, many team members expressed concern about this approach and sought to subvert these demands through the exertion of temporal agency. Community mental health nurse (CMHN) Leslie, among others, articulated the potential for 'discharge deaths' and consequently furtively delayed discharging service users from his caseload where he identified potential concerns around a lack of social support. Similarly, Evelyn described 'fudging things' with the Trust in terms of organisational targets in order to ensure she could continue to provide support to service user Harriet. In another example, social worker Yvonne, in her approved mental health professional (AMHP) role, described refusing to certify community treatment order (CTO) forms where she considered psychiatrists to be using this measure in ways that contravened service users' rights.

In addition to these individual, micro-level forms of resistance, more collective and explicitly political practices oriented to meso-level community, social movement and trade union structures were also visible. Leslie noted the influence on his practice of campaigning organisations such as the Hearing Voices Network, the Soteria Network and the Campaign to Abolish the Schizophrenia Label. For Leslie, these and wider interventions by service user movements had played an important role in reframing service user–practitioner power relationships and succeeded in strengthening the challenge to biomedical reductionism in the field.

In another meso-level example, Roger articulated shared interests between workers and service users in the quality of services. This began to evolve towards cross-sectional campaigning alliances between mental health workers, their trade union and service users, through nascent links between UNISON representatives and service user activists. These incipient cross-sectional alliances raised issues such as cuts to services and staffing and were visible around the Walk-In service closure and coordinated challenges to senior managers on the Trust Board. The possibility of meso-level alliances across occupational boundaries, and with service users, was also apparent in a lobby against cuts within the Trust, organised by local anti-austerity activists and attended by service users, and health and social workers.

Alternatives to biomedical residualism: social perspectives and relational goods

The findings presented here and across the fieldwork chapters suggest a continuing identification among many practitioners and service users with social perspectives and relational approaches. However, in this section, I will explore the tension between what I will characterise as the 'thin' conception of social perspectives in neoliberal social inclusion agendas, for instance (neo)recovery, and the 'thick' conceptions of the 'social' visible in the situated social-relational practices and ethico-political orientations enacted by practitioners and discussed in the preceding section. The notion of 'relational goods' will be introduced in order to underpin this distinction.

Contemporary mental health policy and practice is commonly framed in terms of social inclusion (Spandler, 2007). The 'social' constructed in this neoliberal imaginary mobilises powerful progressive and liberatory rhetorics to criticise (with justification) the paternalism and oppressive bureaucracy of preceding (Keynesian and earlier) welfare settlements, but offers only a thin, marketised articulation of this concept in its place (Ferguson, 2007; Beresford, 2016). Core neoliberal inclusion interventions such as neorecovery, personalisation, brief therapies and 'work cure' initiatives limit conceptions of the 'social' to short-term interpersonal encounters that operate mainly to responsibilise the actions of the individual (Brown and Manning, 2018). Furthermore, emergent informational systems and individualising logics and strategic directional tendencies in this neoliberal setting act as a further constraint on more thoroughgoing socially and relationally embedded activities and perspectives. However, this raises the question of the basis on which to distinguish between what I will characterise as 'thin' and 'thick' conceptions of the social (and relational) in mental health services.

Applying the principles of relational realism to this organisational setting enables clarification on this issue. Social interactions between people (as individual or collective subjects) have emergent properties with particular causal potentialities. Under certain conditions, this emergent effect may manifest as a 'relational good' that is mutually produced and experienced by subjects who are in a non-instrumentally motivated relation with each other. The term 'good' is defined here in political philosophy terms, as 'ethically desirable states/behaviours', for example, the common good, rather than goods as products or commodities (Donati, 2016). The emergence of such relational goods requires enabling conditions, and particularly integral to this are reciprocal, symmetrical (that is, non-hierarchical and non-coerced) and non-market relations. Examples of relational goods include trust between people, cooperation between residents in a neighbourhood, bottom-up collaboration in social networks and forms of peer and mutual support.

In health and social care settings, the creation of relational goods requires the development of an egalitarian context of interpersonal interaction to foster trust, cooperation and reciprocity (Sheaff and Pilgrim, 2006). A democratic and dialogical atmosphere between practitioners and service users then has the potential to enable generative and reparative forms of sociability (Donati and Archer, 2015). Examples might include the development of user-led and peer support services (Beresford, 2016), or dialogical and systemic therapeutic approaches such as Open Dialogue.

However, there are a number of barriers to democratic and dialogical social interaction and therefore the emergence of relational goods in mental health services. These include power asymmetries underpinned by legislative frameworks, and hierarchical user–professional relations reinforcing paternalism and other gendered and racialised forms of oppression. These generate forms of epistemic injustice that marginalise and silence service user perspectives and deny participation (Newbigging and Ridley, 2018). Consequently, the potential for emergent relational goods is undermined by 'enforced relationality' or 'relational authoritarianism' in mental health work (Donati and Archer, 2015). This refers to the outcomes of relational interventions that are prescribed within legal frameworks, for example CTOs, or those framed by the unequal structural positioning of participants and attendant social and epistemic inequalities. Thus, while Donati and Archer's (2015) framework highlights the kinds of organisational innovations and reforms necessary to engender relational goods in mental health services, it also foregrounds the significant and continuous threat to their emergence and cultivation posed by market and top-down bureaucratic welfare policy mechanisms.

The implication of this is that the development of authentically social perspectives within the mental health system requires attention to two dimensions. First, purportedly 'social' interventions at the micro/meso level of mental health service provision must be assessed in terms of not only their form but also their content and scope, that is, whether or not they generate relational goods and for whom. Second, any discussion of relational goods necessarily implicates the wider sociopolitical conditions of possibility for their emergence, including the forms of individual and collective agency involved in their generation.

By the first of these criteria, neoliberal 'social' approaches that orient around the responsible individual citizen-consumer (Clarke et al, 2007) fail to recognise the relational interdependencies at the service and community level that are essential to fostering lived experiences of (grassroots) recovery.[1] In contrast, practice initiatives such as My Story and the community work of Farooq involve the co-creation of dialogical and democratic social-relational spaces that offer possibilities for collective engagements that go beyond individualised and transactional social practices, and offer participatory orientations that address and challenge epistemic injustices. This relational approach thus offers clearer ontological criteria for defining social perspectives in mental health: 'thick' relationality; a focus on dialogical democracy and epistemic justice; and an orientation to wider communities, collectives and environments.

Meanwhile, the second consideration draws our attention to the structural and agential conditions necessary for the creation of such social and relational goods. As Chapters 2 and 6 suggest, while these can still develop in the interstices of services under contemporary capitalism, the neoliberalising welfare state generally remains a hostile setting for social-relational practices. The collective agency of senior managers has embedded marketised and risk-oriented organisational structures and created a service environment in which the interleaving of informational mechanisms and market logics has generated strategic directional tendencies towards biomedical residualism and custodial paternalism that constitute a powerful barrier to the emergence of social-relational welfare spaces and interventions.

Nonetheless, a countervailing tendency towards ethico-political professionalism mobilised through forms of individual and collective agency by practitioners, alongside and in combination with the agency of service users, ensured that fragments of relationality remained visible in the CMHT, although even these limited spaces came under increasing pressure within the RRT.

Situational logics and directional tendencies in mental health services: theoretical and practical implications

The preceding section has explained attempts to preserve social-relational spaces and how clearer conceptions of 'thick' social approaches may assist with these agential endeavours. Nonetheless, as the study has illustrated, dominant situational logics and strategic directional tendencies have significantly constrained social-relational practices. Biomedically oriented perspectives and interventions endure and remain integral within mental health services in spite of policy and organisational shifts. In the first part of this final section of the chapter, I seek to illustrate the strengths of the situational logics approach as an explanatory account of this continued prominence of the biomedical through comparison with alternative perspectives. In the second part, I foreground the agential interventions (predominantly by senior management) that have promoted and maintained the conditions sustaining dominant situational logics and directional tendencies. I then conclude by identifying collective agents with the capacity to challenge and transcend these dominant logics and tendencies, and thereby create a new ecological niche more suited to alternative social-relational forms of provision.

Prominent theoretical explanations for the enduring profile of biomedical models in mental health services include the identification of institutional inertia generated by professional socialisation in interaction with hospital-based organisational routines (Rogers and Pilgrim, 2001, p 180), or the role of enduring practice modalities that create a biomedical professional 'habitus' (Brodwin, 2011). However, while these offer useful insights, they represent only a partial explanation. Instead, I will argue that the situational logics approach, and its delineation of multiple interacting layers, offers a more thoroughgoing explanatory account of the persistence of biomedical approaches and concomitant marginalisation of social perspectives.

Understanding the endurance of biomedical perspectives

The findings of this study suggest that, while professional socialisation, habitus and routinisation may play a role in shaping models-in-use by practitioners under certain limited conditions, institutional procedures and occupational socialisation are insufficient to operate as a hydraulic pressure generating adherence to particular practice modalities or professional ideologies. There is not one occupational group engaged with a single policy framework in the mental health system (if that were the case then a model of hydraulic socialisation might be plausible). Instead, from the community care era and particularly since the emergence of the neoliberal settlement, this domain has been constituted by a complex array of organisational and policy structures. Within this, a range of occupational groups, service users and senior managers informed by multiple ideational frameworks interact in a sometimes complementary but frequently conflictual manner.

As practitioners navigate these sedimented and contested organisational environments, they find that their 'habits of thinking' (Sayer 2011), that is, the procedural and/or occupational practices and ideas into which they have been socialised, may be either reinforced or challenged by the situational logics and directional tendencies that they encounter. In other words, contextual demands provide 'reasons for action' that orient mental health workers' evaluations of which models to deploy. Thus, it is ultimately situational logics and the directional tendencies they generate that shape (but do not determine) their activity by creating contextually situated pressures and rationales that foreground certain practices and models-in-use and not others. The ideas and practices foregrounded in this way may or may not be associated with a practitioner's particular professional background and socialisation. Consequently, practitioners may enthusiastically, habitually or reluctantly align with these logics and tendencies. Moreover, as agents are always 'sovereign artificers', they may also reject and resist pressures to orient to them if they are willing to pay the opportunity costs (Archer, 1995).

This section illustrates some of these theoretical claims by presenting scenarios from the fieldwork and returning to examples from preceding chapters. In doing so I seek to show why accounts informed by hydraulic socialisation are insufficient to explain developments in this setting. I identify the strengths of an EM approach in comparison with alternatives, by demonstrating the necessity of an account that acknowledges the multiple logics between which practitioners (and service users and carers) navigate. I then conclude with reflections on the explanatory value of the stratified account of agency and orientation to class and broader social struggles offered by EM.

The notion of hydraulic socialisation, in this context, is the assumption that knowledge and practice can be straightforwardly reconfigured through the implementation of new top-down policy frameworks or redesigned labour processes. The earlier chapters have indicated how neoliberal policy makers and senior managers have sought to 'hydraulically' reconfigure organisational and professional cultures through processes such as the metric regimes of NPM. Mechanisms oriented to performance management and implemented via information and communication technologies (ICTs) have sought to procedurally embed hierarchical structural dynamics in institutional routines and inculcate organisational dispositions, thereby limiting the discretionary spaces available to professionals (Mutch, 2019).

A scenario from the fieldwork involving assistant director Terry illustrates this. Terry attended a CMHT meeting one week to present the initial SLM restructure proposals to Southville CMHT team members. Terry framed these changes in terms of the potential achievement of better service user outcomes and levels of satisfaction. Social worker Ruth and CMHN Kath captured a general mood of scepticism when they explained to him how hard it was to be person-centred (that is, to deploy a values-based social-relational approach) when predominant target-driven requirements to input and manage data reduced contact with service users.

Terry replied: "But the service needs to be person-centred or we won't meet our targets" and shortly after added, "regardless of the admin, we need to prioritise care. Person-centred is the dominant philosophy."

EM's mode of analysis offers support for CMHT team members' sceptical position. The target regime mechanism advocated by Terry is extremely unlikely to hydraulically generate a person-centred outcome because it decouples the realisation of these cultural emergent properties (person-centred values) from the structural contexts that may enable (or constrain) their articulation. The paradox of the neoliberalisation of services, noted earlier, is that the very market-oriented mechanisms deployed (purportedly) to improve accountability and deliver 'social inclusion' undermine the conditions for the trusting interpersonal engagements necessary to generate relational goods and thereby achieve those goals. The other prominent policy and organisational agendas in this setting, including informational demands, risk actuarialism (via biomedical approaches) and responsibilisation (Brown and Baker, 2012), overdetermine social inclusion imperatives, undermining the generation of relational goods and producing instead directional tendencies towards biomedical residualism. Regardless of the intentions informing the design of these 'person-centred targets' by managers or those underpinning their implementation by individual practitioners, the market-oriented informational practice systems of neoliberalism offer an ecological niche more congruent with biomedical residualism than social-relational approaches.

While this example refers to attempts at top-down organisational socialisation, the critique of hydraulic assumptions can equally be applied to professional socialisation. Whether or not practitioners are able to orient to the models and practices associated with their professional background and socialisation is dependent on the context, and the extent to which the logics and directional tendencies within which they are enmeshed enable or constrain the articulation of these approaches. This means that, in practice, mental health workers move strategically between various models/practices, those into which they have been professionally socialised but also other frameworks, according to the institutional demands placed on them and attendant spaces for discretion. The situational logics approach delineates the contours of agential possibility that operate to shape (although not determine) the models and practices available. The next section will draw on examples to illustrate this process.

In Chapter 5 we encountered social worker Filipe's shift from a social to a biomedical frame for understanding service user Alistair's experiences of mental distress. Crucial to understanding Filipe's shift in his conceptual lens were the exigencies of the organisational context. When Alistair was not in immediate mental health crisis (that is, during what practitioners tended to refer to as a 'stable' phase), Filipe had a greater room for discretionary manoeuvre. Although the dominant logic and directional tendency within this context is biomedical residualism, he chose to align instead as far as possible with a social-relational approach, mobilising a systemic-therapeutic approach that accorded more closely with his professional socialisation as a social worker and his ethical commitments. However, when Alistair entered what was regarded as an 'acute' phase of distress, the demands of the risk-averse organisational culture within the Trust required Filipe to adopt a more medicalised risk management strategy. In this context, his identification with the professional interest group of social work was outweighed by the potential costs associated with failure to adhere to Trust risk policy frameworks. Thus, although risk management policy did not act as a 'hydraulic pressure' on Filipe to conform to this medicalised approach, it nonetheless exerted conditioning effects on him through, on the one hand, the provision of a biomedical rationale for changing to a more interventionist 'treatment' orientation but, on the other, the potential opportunity costs if he declined to do so, in the form of the negative consequences of the 'inquiry culture' and potential disciplinary action for his career trajectory as well as the expectations associated with his deputy manager role. Consequently, Filipe reoriented to a strategic directional tendency of custodial paternalism in the form of a biomedical orientation combined with custodial risk management.

Further instances of this phenomenon gave support to the notion of these logics and directional tendencies as a broad and durable feature of this organisational context regardless of the professional background of those enmeshed within them. For instance, CMHN Bill described moving along a continuum between social and more biomedically oriented perspectives according to contextual demands. As he noted,

'You'll get [mental health nurses] who are totally aligned with the ... medical model and you'll get people at the other end of the spectrum ... the empowering of service users and the voice-hearing movement ... The rest of us are all on that continuum somewhere and I guess some of us move, it's not static ... It's probably the amount of distress that the person's experiencing ... plus risk that ... gauges where I'm [positioned].'

Thus, like social worker Filipe, Bill shifted from a social-relational towards a more biomedical approach when issues of risk were perceived to have escalated.

This tendency was also visible in situations where professional and personal epistemologies were seen to be in conflict. An example is the divergence between CMHN Abbie and psychiatrist James over the recommendation for Manu to be placed in a forensic setting, perhaps reflecting different ethical orientations at the personal level. However, when issues of risk were regarded as escalating then their recommendations and actions converged around custodialism.

Similarly, social worker Farooq often described divergent perspectives between himself and psychiatrists regarding the latter's over-medicalisation of service users' concerns. However there were, increasingly, convergences underpinned by organisational pressures. In a scenario first introduced in Chapter 2, Farooq recounted carrying out a Mental Health Act (MHA) assessment in his role as an AMHP following a 'Friday afternoon' referral (this implies defensive risk management before a weekend service closure on the part of the referrer). Farooq and the two psychiatrists involved had reluctantly arrived at a decision to admit the service user to an inpatient ward under section 3 of the MHA in order to 'cover backs'. This illustrates both the existence of interprofessional divergences between social work and psychiatry, but also increasing convergence in their practices in the context of institutional requirements for prudential risk management (a directional tendency of custodial paternalism). These examples all suggest some room for discretion when service users were perceived to be in a 'stable' phase (where divergent professional epistemologies may be more visible), but this was significantly more limited during the so-called 'acute' phase, when action was reoriented to align with dominant situational logics and directional tendencies.

This also illustrates the 'layered' and sedimented composition of these institutional contexts, where archaic forms such as custodialism co-exist alongside long-established relational and newer informational systems, practices and temporalities, with practitioners reflexively navigating between these according to the requirements and demands of the context. These variegated temporal orders and associated forms of temporal agency were particularly visible in the transition from CMHT to RRT. While, in the CMHT, informational demands had increasingly encroached on, and squeezed out, relational casework in care coordination through reductions in porous time, practitioners still maintained some potential to exert discretion and carve out relational spaces in their care coordination work (for example, Leslie's 'tree of life' work with service user Ray). In the RRT, by contrast, the practice space of care coordination itself was increasingly marginalised and replaced by duty work. Thus, the restructured labour process did not just squeeze out but increasingly foreclosed the possibility for practitioners to engage in longer-term relational casework. In this way the shift from relational to informational that emerged during the CMHT era is extended and deepened in the RRT. The intensification of strenuous welfarism through a predominantly informational labour process impinged on participants through the changing temporal orders of mental health practice and the dissonances thereby generated.

Practitioners and service users responded in diverse ways to the various logics, directional tendencies and attendant temporal dynamics associated with them. For practitioners, there was pressure to conform to the demands generated by this performative informational culture, which seeks to reconstruct the subjectivity of the mental health worker as a 'quantified self' (Moore, 2018) to meet the demands of the 'green dashboard'. Such processes generated a 'hysteresis effect', which describes tensions associated with attempts to continue to implement established forms of professional practice while changes in the service environment create challenges in doing so (Brodwin, 2011). Practitioners responded in different ways to this effect. For Abbie, a sense of tension and frustration arose as informational temporal pressures collided with a slower custodial temporality, and as a result she sought to accelerate Manu's move into forensic services. In contrast, while the pressures at the interface between social-relational and neoliberal informational temporalities generated anxiety for Leslie too, he sought to cultivate a recalcitrant nonchalance, resolving to slow discharges of 'backburner clients'. Kath also asserted temporal agency by carving out slower social-relational engagements within the space of the depot clinic. Thus, both accommodation and resistance to the dominant (informational) temporal order were visible.

Another significant effect of dominant situational logics and directional tendencies under neoliberalism is the reinforcing of a psychocentrist orientation, with the individual level construed as the limit of the explanatory horizon in relation to mental distress. This narrows the possibilities among practitioners for conceptualising the psychosocial effects of, and collective responses to, social structural and institutional processes such as exploitation, discrimination, oppression and stigmatisation. These lacunae have significant implications for service users. For instance, this was visible in James and Abbie's evaluations of Manu's levels of responsibility and risk in Chapter 4, and their custodial and biomedical responses, and the marginalisation of structural and institutional conceptualisations of the role of racism.[2] Similarly, the role of social factors related to workplace stressors remained somewhat marginal in the reflections by Filipe and James on Alistair's experiences of distress.

Dominant situational logics and directional tendencies not only individualise social experiences, but also tend to 'squeeze out' the spaces for engagement with alternative ethico-political and social-relational conceptions and practices (that is, countervailing directional tendencies of ethico-political professionalism). The informational pressures and temporal constraints encountered by Farooq are an example. These meant he was no longer able to engage in the community work practices with the local British Pakistani community that had previously succeeded in focusing the attention of the Trust and team on addressing institutional forms of racism, discrimination and exclusion faced by this group. Farooq felt that, as a result of his withdrawal from this role due to organisational demands, the unmet needs of community members and institutionalised barriers to services had increased. He also felt this had lowered levels of recognition within the Trust and among practitioners of these institutional barriers and their effects for this particular community.

Agents of change: from role action to collective agency and alliances

The account developed in the previous section has focused on the reproduction of the organisational environment of mental health services through dominant situational logics and directional tendencies. Moreover, it adopted a critical stance on the effects of these, arguing that they generate relational absences associated with harmful consequences. I will now return to the theme of *countervailing* logics and tendencies introduced in the first part of the chapter. I will extend this discussion by examining forms of human agency, both those associated with institutional reproduction but also more significantly those underpinning the potential for transformational interventions to challenge relational absences.

There have been significant changes in the prevailing power relations within the mental health system since the early 1990s. As Archer (1995, p 152) argues, structural 'transformation is rooted in determinate conflicts between identifiable groups who find themselves in particular positions with particular interests to advance or defend'. Up until the 1990s, the capitalist state delegated the management of mental healthcare to the profession of psychiatry either as the dominant (in the early 20th-century hospital system) or leading profession in a multiprofessional context (during the later 20th-century iterations of community care). However, since the implementation of neoliberal mental healthcare reform, there has been a shift from medical to managerial dominance under neoliberalism (Ramon, 2008). The establishment of a pre-eminent position for a cadre of senior managers has destabilised and reshaped other longstanding determinate conflicts within this institutional arena (for instance, service user–professional and interprofessional),[3] as well as generating new ones.

One significant example of this is the rise to prominence of clinical psychology as medical dominance has come under challenge. Key elements of psychology's professional knowledge base and interventions have proven highly compatible with the restructured ecological niche of welfare and mental health services under neoliberalism.[4] In Chapter 7, psychiatrist James described this as a significant threat to his own profession's health and status. However, as he later observed, interprofessional competition and conflict deflected from a more fundamental division under neoliberalism, that between "workers and bosses" in the context of intensifying managerial dominance. For CMHN Roger too, institutional challenges were occasionally articulated in terms of interagency/interprofessional tensions even though he generally sought to foreground solidarity between occupational groups in his trade union work within the Trust.

This highlights the utility of the theoretical distinction in the EM framework between *agent* (the person's position within, in this example, a system of class stratification) and *institutional actor* (based on occupational background and attendant normative role expectations). This stratified conception of the person enables analysis of the mutual interplay between workplace role and broader personal (for example, class, gender, racialised, sexual) identities and the sociopolitical implications of this for individual and collective action within this institutional setting. The frustrations articulated by James and Roger (that were shared by many other practitioners in the study) typically followed an interprofessional contour, foregrounding their *role actor* identities as psychiatrist, nurse or social worker. Moreover, the fragmentation of National Health Service (NHS) trade unions, the representative institutions of workers as (collective) 'agents', into separate 'service groups' for health and social services, has reinforced these tendencies and exacerbated the barriers to coordinated action by mental health workers across professional groups. However, as both Roger and James acknowledged, interprofessional disputes represent a refractory process that has tended to obscure more politically salient class-based shifts in organisational power relations within the NHS. The implication of such a shift is that potential solutions in the form of collective agency (for example, trade union or social movement mobilisation) are thereby opened up.

Another important determinate contour of conflict within the context of mental health services is that between service users and professionals. As the occupational group most strongly historically associated with policy mechanisms and technologies of coercive social control of users, psychiatry has been a particular focus of this tension.[5] In Chapter 3, several service users discussed opposition or resistance to forms of psychiatric control. For example, Harriet described feeling compelled to conceal her decision not to adhere to her prescribed antipsychotic medication due to fear of the potential for psychiatric responses characterised by compulsion and deprivation of liberty. As Harriet noted, service users have mobilised to challenge these oppressive experiences, and this social movement activity, which first emerged in its contemporary form in the wake of wider liberation struggles of the 1960s to 1970s, represents a shift from diffuse forms of primary (individual) action to new forms of collective mobilisation (that is, collective agency) by service users/survivors (Spandler, 2006; Survivors History Group, 2011; Beresford, 2016). This new agential collectivity (the service user/survivor movement) has therefore taken its place alongside other collective agents whose activity is directed towards maintenance or change in the mental health system, such as professional interest groups and trade unions.

It is important to recognise, however, that while the relationship between users and professionals is commonly perceived to be characterised by conflicting interests, this reflects a 'role actor' lens of analysis. Once this lens is widened beyond institutional role action to include *social agency* (based on interests arising from pre-structured societal resource distributions), then other actual and potential interrelational permutations come into view. These include both contradictory opposed interests *and* potential complementarities. For instance, NHS and social services senior managers have sought to highlight service user–professional conflicts over paternalism in order to develop strategic alignments with service user collective agents. They have done so by promoting neoliberal consumerism through policy agendas such as personalisation (Ferguson, 2007), or rationalising neoliberal target cultures within services as a means to promote social inclusion (for example, assistant director Terry's comment about person-centred targets). However, the fieldwork chapters have illustrated the limits of this top-down strategy for achieving 'thick' relational forms of support. Moreover, these chapters illustrated significant incompatibilities and potential for conflict between senior management and service users (as collective agents) arising from the implementation of a neoliberal austerity agenda.

Conversely, some groups of progressive and radical professionals have aligned with service user-led campaigns, for instance the challenge by service users to the management-imposed and austerity-related closure of the valued Walk-In service. Others have sought to implement forms of dialogical democratisation from below (for example, the worker–service user co-facilitation of My Story) that challenge paternalism. Both examples suggest a tendency, noted at the start of the chapter, for both workers and service users to value more comprehensive services oriented to longer-term forms of social-relational support. Herein reside potential shared interests between these two collectivities that offer a basis for forms of joint mobilisation between labour and survivor movements (Moth and McKeown, 2016).

Moreover, as the study has shown, neoliberal reforms and the dominant situational logics arising from them represent major obstacles to realising these more social-relational and ethico-politically informed responses to mental distress. Consequently, the shared ground on which such service user–worker cross-sectional alliances might be built is likely to include demands for 'thick' social approaches and ethico-politically sensitive services. By the latter I mean the democratisation of forms of support, combining expertise by experience and expertise by profession[6] within egalitarian structures, and services strongly oriented to recognising the role of harms associated with class inequalities, exploitation and various forms of oppression and to challenging these (Moth and McKeown, 2016).[7] Joint mobilisations around such demands would represent a challenge to biomedical residualism and custodial paternalism and thus offer transformative potential for the reorientation of services towards social-relational alternatives.

This reframes the primary tensions in services from 'role' conflicts between service users and practitioners to contestation between the agential collectivities of senior management on one side, and labour and service user movements on the other. Alignments of the latter kind are not automatic, and there can be significant barriers to their development. Nonetheless, as the book has highlighted, there are possibilities for 'cross-sectional alliances' (that is, forms of class-based collective agency) that bring mental health workers from different occupational groups together alongside service users in forms of collective action to reshape and democratise this sphere. Although these remain, in a general sense, an emergent potential yet to be fully actualised within this setting, nascent small-scale signs of such alliances are nonetheless visible (McKeown et al, 2014; Sedgwick, 2015; Moth and McKeown, 2016).

In summary, my contention has been that the value of theorising situational logics and directional tendencies within a wider EM approach is that it enables analysis of the structural, cultural and agential dynamics that shape how practitioners and service users make sense of and respond to lived experiences of mental distress within this organisational domain. An understanding of these logics and tendencies enables recognition of the complex alignment of features that underpin dominant ideas and practices within neoliberalising services. However, it also enables identification of the forms of collective agency and alliances through which contemporary conditions and their dominant situational logics might be transcended. These forms of agency offer possibilities to reshape and transform the prevailing forms of knowledge and practice through the creation of alternative participatory, egalitarian and democratic forms of support.

Conclusion

In this concluding chapter, I will begin with a brief review of the theoretical orientation of the book and its core arguments. Having done so, I will then consider the sociopolitical implications of these arguments for policy and practice within the mental health system, the wider welfare state and beyond.

The book has argued that in the context of marketised and digitalising mental health service reconfigurations, emergent situational logics and associated directional tendencies such as biomedical residualism have become dominant. While proponents of the strengthening of the market/digital nexus within organisations claim that these reforms deliver increased efficiencies (Eubanks, 2018; Trittin-Ulbrich et al, 2021), the findings from this study have identified significant negative impacts for service users and practitioners. The transition from community care to neoliberal modalities of practice has promoted virtuality, audit-driven and surface-oriented interventions and relegated embodied co-presence to the margins of the work, restricting opportunities for the development of trust and compassion. This shift from relational approaches to informational practices has, consequently, undermined the contextual mediators of such qualities in the form of relationships, cultures and healing environments (Spandler and Stickley, 2011).

For service users these have produced metric-driven harms in so far as these constrain opportunities for the kinds of interpersonal relational engagements that strengthen processes of (grassroots) recovery. Similarly, for practitioners, digitalisation has facilitated the neoliberal restructuring of the labour process (Moore et al, 2018) and increased managerial control (Reid, 2003). This, as the findings have shown, has resulted in both work intensification and a reduction of discretionary spaces for relationship-based interactions with service users. Because of these interrelated processes, opportunities to practise in ways commensurate with professional and ethical preferences have been limited (Worrall et al, 2010), leading to frustrations and 'ethical stress' (Fenton, 2015). However, while, in many cases, practitioners have adjusted to these imposed limitations, challenges to them are also visible, ranging from 'work arounds' (Lammi, 2021) such as adapting relational practices to informational environments, or working after hours to create temporal openings for relational casework, to more overt forms of ethico-political intervention (Mather and Seifert, 2017; Karsten, 2021).

This confluence of informational restructuring, notions of user responsibility and older discourses of risk under neoliberalism has generated powerful directional tendencies that constrain relational spaces of support and foreground restrictive and medicalised practices. Consequently, the legitimacy of mental health services has been undermined for many service users and allies, and there have been increasing calls for a participatory and democratising transformation of this setting (Beresford, 2016; Spandler and McKeown, 2017). The findings of this study have pointed to support for these kinds of normative-relational transformations among many mental health workers as well as service users. However, at least three necessary dimensions of any such social-relational reorientation have been identified: 'thick' relationality; epistemic equality/dialogical democracy; and collective and community focus.

As Chapter 9 noted, the creation of relational goods within mental health services is highly dependent on certain enabling conditions. The 'thin' relationality and time-limited nature of much provision in contemporary mental health services can undermine this goal, as can the instrumentalising of relational interactions. In contrast, thick relationality involves longer-term mutual forms of social interaction and support, characterised by reciprocal and non-hierarchical relations. Such shifts from paternalist practices to collaborative and co-productive engagements between practitioners and service users require transformations involving the dismantling of the epistemic priority accorded dominant groups and the development of structures of dialogical democracy[1] (Beresford, and Carr, 2018; Carrigan, 2018).

A further crucial transformative dimension is the shift from an individualist to a collectivist orientation. Neoliberal policy has tended to valorise independence rather than interdependence. This has reconfigured services around individualised forms of support and away from community approaches and collective forms of provision (Jordan, 2007), resulting in an agenda of enforced individualism (Roulstone and Morgan, 2009). As a result, relational spaces of collective and community support have been increasingly marginalised in statutory mental health services, as the example of the closure of the Walk-In at Southville illustrates. However, as Klinenburg (2018) argues, social infrastructure in the form of buildings and social spaces where people can interact and offer mutual support plays a crucial role in creating the kinds of 'affective community spaces' and 'healing communities' that increase wellbeing by reducing isolation and strengthening social connection (Warner et al, 2013; Van Os et al, 2019).

However, as well as defining the necessary contexts of and for relationality, there is also the question of the forms of agency by which such social-relational environments might be realised. Such agency has long been evident among service user/survivor movements, in the form of struggles for the democratisation of forms of mental health provision through a more fundamentally inclusive and participatory orientation (Beresford, 2016; Beresford and Carr, 2018). Alongside this, democratising impulses have also been visible among some radical practitioners. Earlier forms of radical mental health practice such as institutional psychotherapy (identified with Tosquelles and Frantz Fanon), therapeutic communities and Italian democratic psychiatry were all based on challenging the sedimented, repressive institutions of psychiatry. These projects involved, in diverse ways, democratising relations between recipients and providers of services within and beyond the organisational context of the psychiatric hospital (Foot, 2015; Robcis, 2016; Wall, 2018; Garrett, 2020). Despite the considerable challenges posed by the neoliberalisation of the welfare state, some signs of aspiration towards a more radical professionalism remain visible both in this study, and more widely in the welfare professions (Ferguson, 2017b).

So what, then, are the political implications of these findings? I will conclude the chapter and book by identifying two in particular. The first is that there is significant incompatibility between social-relational, democratic forms of mental health support and processes of the neoliberalisation of the welfare state. Second, as a consequence of the first, it will be necessary for collective agents to engage in more fundamentally transformative forms of resistance if participatory and relational forms of mental health provision are to be realised. While such politically engaged activities were relatively marginal during the fieldwork, potentialities for collective action and mobilisation were nonetheless discernible in this setting, as Chapter 9 noted. Moreover, the study's theoretical lens offers a potential means to conceptualise the legacy of earlier progressive settlements from which a contemporary reimagining of provision might be forged, and I will now turn to the latter.

As we have seen, Marx argued that certain organisational 'remnants' may embody progressive political possibilities in their 'form', even while divestment of some residual regressive elements of 'content' may be necessary (Harootunian, 2015, p 54).[2] One such potentially progressive *form* in relation to mental health services is Keynesian welfarist 'community care', which highlighted universalism, social equality and relational principles. However, the *content* of this model was, in practice, undermined by underfunding, the reproduction of structural discrimination in its delivery mechanisms in relation to gender, 'race', sexuality and other social divisions, and a paternalist orientation towards service users (Ferguson et al, 2002; Beresford, 2016). From the 1980s onwards, these shortcomings enabled the New Right to mobilise a 'progressive neoliberal' critique of Keynesian welfarism evoking principles of 'choice' and 'freedom' (Harris, 2018; Cummins, 2020). However, as Ferguson et al (2002) and Beresford (2016) have argued, elements of the post-war welfare settlement delivered significant progressive social reforms, even while their transformative and participatory potentials failed to be fully realised. However, by bringing together the liberatory energies and democratising impulses of contemporary social movements challenging oppression (such as the service user/survivor, disabled people's,

Black Lives Matter, MeToo and lesbian, gay, bisexual, trans and queer [LGBTQ] movements) with the structural influence of labour movements demanding workplace justice, possibilities for further transformative advances in universal and egalitarian welfare remain.

This argument should not, however, be read as an evocation of nostalgia for a lost 'golden age' of community mental health services that existed in the pre-neoliberal era, even though, on one occasion, that very phrase was used directly by a practitioner to contrast earlier iterations of the Community Mental Health Team (CMHT) with the damage wrought by current neoliberal reform. This is because, notwithstanding the emergence of some progressive relational approaches during the community care era, this period was characterised by what Spandler (2016) has called 'psychiatric abuse' in mainstream services, ranging from institutionalisation and iatrogenesis to paternalism and oppression.[3] The progressive elements of Keynesian community care do, though, represent a kernel of future potentialities, unrealised possibilities on which more egalitarian and participatory understandings of and responses to mental distress might be built.

However, which of these emergent possibilities, progressive or regressive, will prevail in mental health services is shaped both by the structural potentialities of the environment and also, crucially, by the political and ideational responses of those within it. In other words, whatever social structural potentialities may inhere in this 'specifically political present' (Bensaïd, 2002, pp 71–72), the outcomes are contingent upon the (political) activity of individual but crucially also collective agents within services and society.

Although very small in scale, the nascent challenges to neoliberalisation described in this study hint at potentials both to go beyond institutional constraints to relationality within the mental health system, but at the same time to contribute to the sociopolitical contestation of broader distributive inequalities and forms of oppression at the societal level. In so far as madness and mental distress constitute materially structured lived experiences underpinned by social, economic and political inequalities, such sociopolitical challenges have an important role to play in addressing both the iniquitous determinants of distress and their consequences (Muntaner and Geiger-Brown, 2006; Ferguson, 2017a; Stanford et al, 2017).

Thus, the emerging forms of collective agency in social and labour movements have potential significance not only as an expression of democratising impulses and participatory possibilities in wider society but also within service user–worker relationships and welfare state institutions (Beresford, 2016, pp 264–265; Lethbridge, 2019). They point to possibilities for the creation of more relational forms of social and community support but also to more thoroughly collective and political conceptions of recovery itself (Dillon, 2011; Harper and Speed, 2012; Brown and Manning, 2018).

Such conceptions highlight the limitations of an individualised lens for understanding and responding to mental distress. They also foreground the necessity and urgency of sociopolitical transformations to transcend the toxic psychosocial environment generated by neoliberal capitalism.

Appendix: methodology

This appendix will provide a brief overview of the study's methodology. The broad aims of the study were to explore the impact of policy and organisational reforms implemented within Community Mental Health Teams (CMHTs) on the articulation and negotiation of differing conceptualisations of mental distress. Participant observation utilising a 'reflexive ethnography' approach (Davies, 2008) formed the primary research method for this particularistic (small-group) ethnographic study. Additional methods included semi-structured qualitative individual and group interviews, and document analysis.

Data collection was carried out in two phases. Having obtained ethical clearance from the relevant NHS Research Ethics Committee,[1] an initial eight-week pilot study was carried out in a CMHT within a large urban NHS Foundation Trust during 2008. However, it was not possible to continue data collection there for organisational reasons, and so a second team within the same NHS Trust was selected for the full-scale stage of the study. The first full-scale phase of fieldwork was, therefore, carried out between 2009 and 2011. I collected data by immersing myself in the daily routines and functioning of the teams in order to observe everyday practices. The latter included the individual and group casework meetings of practitioners with service users, and multiprofessional fora such as Care Programme Approach (CPA) meetings, inpatient ward rounds and weekly CMHT meetings. In total, I carried out 12 months of data collection utilising participant observation over a three-year period. Following this, I conducted 27 in-depth semi-structured interviews with 19 practitioners based at Southville CMHT and the wider Trust, and eight service users and three carers linked to the CMHT.

During the ethnographic fieldwork, data were recorded in several formats. Scratch notes were handwritten contemporaneously, while at the end of each day detailed field notes and reflective memos were typed up. I audio-recorded and transcribed some meetings and ward rounds, and all individual and group interviews conducted during both phases of the study.

The selection of the fieldwork setting for phase one involved both theoretical and pragmatic considerations. A statutory CMHT was chosen as an appropriate setting to address the research topic because this type of team has been the mainstay of community mental health provision and a number of occupational groups work together within an integrated team framework. This was also a pragmatic choice as I had been employed as a social worker within this particular Trust during the period when access was being negotiated (although had not worked within either of the teams studied).

This raises the issue of field role, that is, how the ethnographer positions the self in the research setting on a continuum from complete participation to complete observation (Hammersley and Atkinson, 2007). In this case, my predominant field role when attending formal team or casework meetings was as an observer because, although data were collected at a Mental Health Trust in which I had formerly worked, I was not employed as a social worker in either of the teams in which the research was conducted. In practice, I engaged in appropriate non-therapeutic social interaction to place participants at ease and interacted when invited to do so. However, in more informal work settings such as the office where practitioners were based, I spent time alongside team members interacting to explore aspects of their work but also engaging in workplace conversations that may or may not be practice related.

By the second phase, the Trust had reconfigured team structures. Consequently, data collection carried out during 2018 and 2019 was with Southville practitioners now working in the Rehabilitation and Recovery (RRT) team, as well as former Southville CMHT workers who had recently left the team or retired. This phase involved one group interview with 10 practitioners, and in-depth semi-structured individual interviews with seven practitioners. Ethical clearance was obtained from Liverpool Hope University Research Ethics Committee.

Unfortunately, resource and time constraints meant I was unable to include service users and carers in the study's second phase and I acknowledge this as a significant limitation of the study. Another limitation is the impact of my identity as a (White) male researcher. A social worker explained to me during phase one that several of the female service users with whom she worked would not be comfortable with observation by a male researcher due to their experience of childhood sexual abuse. This and related factors shaped the demographic characteristics of participants in the study, with a majority of service user participants being male despite my attempts to recruit more female service users. The two case studies in Chapters 4 and 5, both focusing on male service users, reflect this. A third limitation is that due to access issues it was not ultimately possible to interview Manu and his mother as intended. Nonetheless, I have sought to reflect their positions as articulated in meetings observed.

Data analysis was not clearly delineated from other stages of the research process. It remained a continuous focus throughout the fieldwork and write-up during the first phase. I utilised a form of thematic analysis, drawing on Layder's notions of adaptive theory and 'orienting concepts'. This seeks to construct novel theoretical frameworks in the process of ongoing research practice by drawing from aspects of prior theory, general or substantive, in conjunction with theory emerging from data collection and analysis. Furthermore, this approach seeks to formulate links between the level of actors' meaning making and that of the institutional and wider systemic context (Layder, 1993, 1998). The adaptive theoretical framework developed from phase one was revised on the basis of analytic work arising from the second phase of data collection.

All participants in the study have been assigned a pseudonym. A more detailed outline of the study's methodology, during its first phase, is available in Moth (2014).

Notes

Introduction

[1] This is frequently referred to as the 'medical model', which is a somewhat amorphous attribution. Pilgrim et al (2008) trace the emergence of this concept to professional psychiatry's mid-19th-century project to achieve pre-eminence over 'mental disorder' and identify three strands: administrative jurisdiction over madness; a biological causation; and a eugenic consensus about mental abnormality. However, it should be noted that critics of bioreductionism, for instance Engel (1977) who developed the biopsychosocial model, have nonetheless retained the term 'medical model' for their alternative orientation.

[2] The Power Threat Meaning Framework has garnered both support and critique from mental health activists (Grant and Gadsby, 2018; Scheherazade, 2018; Johnstone et al, 2019).

[3] While I have attempted to reflect the contested nature of terminology in this context, I generally use the term 'mental distress' (although also sometimes 'madness') to reflect my own positioning that rejects pathologising categorisations of 'mental illness' and 'mental disorder' (see Sapey et al, 2015, p 6, for further discussion of these debates). While a term such as 'madness' remains controversial, it is increasingly used (reclaimed) in activist and academic contexts, reflecting recent developments such as Mad Studies (Le Francois et al, 2013; Beresford, 2019) and earlier movements such as Mad Pride (Curtis et al, 2000).

[4] The EM approach draws on both the classical Marxist and critical realist traditions, the latter including the sociology of Margaret Archer and philosophy of Roy Bhaskar (Creaven, 2000, 2007). This overarching framework, including the notion of 'situational logics' and 'strategic directional guidance/tendencies', is very briefly introduced in Chapter 1, is mainly implicit in the fieldwork Chapters 2–7, before a more comprehensive overview is provided in Chapter 8.

[5] These include a significant period of mental health crisis experienced by my father during my childhood. They also include my own occasional experiences of mental distress. However, having only used primary and not secondary care mental health services, I do not wish to imply that my own experiences are in any way comparable to the more significant and serious lived experiences of mental distress of service users at Southville Community Mental Health Team (CMHT) and elsewhere. Furthermore, I wish to acknowledge that my personal identity as a White, male researcher positions me socially and institutionally in ways that have influenced my lived experiences and access to resources, and have shaped the conduct and findings of the study.

[6] The PhD study on which this book is (mainly) based was funded for one year by the Centre of Excellence in Interdisciplinary Mental Health (CEIMH) at the University of Birmingham, and then the remaining three years by the Economic and Social Research Council (ESRC). I am extremely grateful to both CEIMH and ESRC for this funding and support.

[7] See the Sedgwick special issue in *Critical and Radical Social Work*, 4(3), November 2016.

[8] See the methodology in the Appendix for a more detailed overview.

[9] I also had some continued informal contact with practitioner participants in 2012 and 2013.

[10] By this time, due to organisational restructuring, this team had been reconfigured as a Rehabilitation and Recovery Team. The implications of these changes will be discussed in detail in Chapter 6.

[11] See the methodology in the Appendix for further detail.

12   The term 'racialised communities' is utilised in the book instead of the more widely used 'Black, Asian and minority ethnic (BAME)' groups in recognition of the limitations of the latter term (Ahmadzadeh, 2021).

Chapter 1

1   This challenges Foucault's (1961) claims of a mid-17th-century 'Great Confinement' across Europe.

2   For instance, the custodialism of Victorian legislation such as the Lunacy Act 1890 (Rogers and Pilgrim, 2001).

3   These drew on earlier eugenic concepts based on highly discriminatory racialised and class hierarchies. These continue to influence contemporary practice in mental health through psychiatric genetics (and 'inherited intelligence' testing in psychology) (Pilgrim, 2008). See Chapter 4 for further discussion on this theme.

4   Although the policy discourse of community care had been present in the 1926 Royal Commission and the Mental Treatment 1930 Act (Pilgrim, 2009).

5   The biopsychosocial model derived from Engel should be differentiated from the biopsychosocial model developed by Waddell and Aylward as part of the UK government's recent welfare reform (and disentitlement) strategy (Shakespeare et al, 2017).

6   The term 'survivor' has become a prominent form of collective self-identification and refers to survival from oppressive psychiatric systems (Beresford, 2012).

7   Due to political resistance and public opposition, the NHS and Community Care Act reforms introduced by the Conservative administration of 1987–92 were unable to deliver wholesale privatisation of the health system (Bartlett and Harrison, 1993).

8   And later, integrated health and social care trusts as provider organisations (Glasby and Tew, 2015).

9   Another important and related dimension of neoliberal reform is *pharmaceuticalisation*, which spans the three modalities of marketisation, consumerism and risk management. Davies (2017) offers a useful take on how pharmaceuticalisation is 'organically attuned' to the aims of neoliberal political economy. Psychopharmaceuticals facilitate the desired affective characteristics of the ideal neoliberal subject, thereby enabling greater labour productivity, and these are more time and cost-effective for employers and governments in treatment and management terms than more expensive relational/therapeutic interventions.

10   This is discussed in more detail in Chapter 4.

Chapter 2

1   Although this is dependent on the availability of such support, which has been limited in the context of austerity-related retrenchment (Moth et al, 2018).

2   One social worker formally consented to involvement in this study but, in practice, did not wish to engage with the study. Although she did not formally withdraw, her data have not been included.

3   The notion of 'old school manager' is used to convey a more consensual style of management in the public sector, associated with less hierarchically structured professions such as social work during the Keynesian era, in contrast to a target-focused 'domination managerialism' under neoliberalism (Evans, 2016). This should be differentiated from the notion of 'old school psychiatrist', sometimes referred to by practitioners and service users, which is intended to evoke a traditional, authoritarian style of practice reflecting medical dominance.

4   Dr James Bryant was generally referred to, and addressed, as James by Southville team members, while service users tended to use the formal title 'Dr Bryant'. In this book, James will be used in most instances, although Dr Bryant where it is appropriate to the

context described. First names were utilised by colleagues and service users to address other Southville practitioners.

[5] A range of medical, pseudo-medical and lay terms were broadly in use by practitioners, service users and others to describe these lived experiences or 'mental states'. For 'stable', alternative terms included "well", "settled" and "chronic" (which had a slightly different inflection). For 'in crisis', alternative descriptors included "relapse", "unwell", "ill", "deteriorating mental health", "psychotic/mood disorder" and (more rarely) "distress". Specific diagnostic categories (for example, depression, bipolar disorder and schizophrenia) were also utilised at times.

[6] Crisis Resolution and Home Treatment Teams (commonly referred to as Crisis Teams) are a form of functionalised team designed to facilitate more intensive daily support of service users in the community than CMHTs are able to provide and to reduce reliance on inpatient care (Burns, 2004).

[7] Some Trusts have recruited former service users to a similar role known as 'peer support worker' (Repper, 2013), although this was not a feature of the CMHT or RRT studied here.

[8] Law and Mooney's (2007) model of 'strenuous welfarism' is a form of labour process theory developed to theorise the effects of neoliberalisation within public sector workers' labour process. This will be described in more detail in Chapter 8.

Chapter 3

[1] The harms associated with this psychiatric temporality of chronicity, and its pathologising and hope-erasing effects, were later challenged by survivor movements and allies (Deegan, 1988; McWade, 2015).

[2] Although this experience of temporal acceleration is context-specific and unevenly socially distributed rather than universal (Sullivan and Gershuny, 2018), it will be argued to be applicable to neoliberalising mental health services.

[3] The tendency towards informational temporalities under neoliberal capitalism is driven by processes of subsumption. This will be described in detail in Chapter 8.

[4] This service was funded by the local authority through partnership agreements with the National Health Service.

[5] This reflects the influence on James's practice of the phenomenology of Louis Sass (2017).

[6] This will be discussed further in Chapter 4.

[7] This approach reflects the situational logic of 'biomedical residualism' described in Chapter 2.

[8] In narrative therapy, 'thin' descriptions are problem-filled labels imposed on people by powerful others, contrasted with 'thick' descriptions, which are preferred stories, based on rich and more comprehensive understandings of the person, rooted in deeper understandings of their histories and identities (White, 1997).

Chapter 4

[1] These services have been given fictional names to protect anonymity.

[2] While this apparently bears some resemblance to James's discussion of developmental issues, I will consider similarities but also important differences when I return to this later.

[3] This quote from James is also used to illustrate the implications of outsourcing described in Chapter 2.

[4] This refers to the homicides of social worker Isabel Schwartz by her former client Sharon Campbell in 1984, and of Jonathan Zito by Christopher Clunis in 1992.

5   Abbie's descriptions of Manu seemed to evoke this stereotype in places.

6   Advocates of eugenics such as Aubrey Lewis were integral to the establishment of the new profession of psychiatry and its organisational centres in the UK, such as the Maudsley Hospital and the Institute of Psychiatry (Fernando, 2017; Gordon-Achebe et al, 2019). As radical psychiatrist Frantz Fanon noted, psychiatry and its knowledge base are deeply implicated in the history of European colonialism as a medium of control of colonised peoples (Harrison, and Burke, 2020). This strengthened psychiatry's perceived legitimacy within state structures at that time. Moreover, the legacy of colonialism is ongoing and extends beyond the Global North. Corporate globalisation has enabled powerful psychiatric and pharmaceutical industry interests to promote and legitimise a new wave of colonisation of the Western biomedical paradigm in the Global South through the top-down Movement for Global Mental Health (Mills, 2014).

7   However, there is also the potential for and sometimes the actuality of ethico-political practices to challenge racism and coloniality within services, professions and society (see Harms-Smith and Nathane, 2018; and Olende, 2020).

Chapter 5

1   Iatrogenic means caused by the activity of the practitioner or treatment itself.

2   However, Healy (2006) goes on to note that the best available evidence demonstrates that suicide risk for those diagnosed with type 1 bipolar disorder is not higher among those who are unmedicated.

3   This model was a forerunner of the more comprehensive duty system that has become integral to the rehabilitation and recovery team (RRT) (see Chapter 6). ART was being trialled in the CMHT during the first phase of fieldwork.

4   However, this serotonin hypothesis is not strongly supported by neuroscientific evidence (Lacasse and Leo, 2005).

5   This is illustrative of the situational logic of biomedical residualism (see Chapter 8).

6   This is a panel convened to hear appeals by service users against MHA detention.

7   A number of CMHT members expressed the view that there were inequalities in terms of greater levels of access to support for more middle-class articulate service users and their families. Filipe's perception that Alistair was prioritised for psychological intervention supports this notion of a class gradient in access to such treatments (Pilgrim, 1997), and the relatively high level of service input with Alistair and Felicity reinforces Clarke et al's (2007) argument that consumer-oriented public services tend to disproportionately benefit those from higher social class backgrounds in terms of resource allocation.

8   While there is a strong relationship between social class and mental health, with poorer people experiencing higher levels of mental distress, it should be noted that there is a complex relationship between socioeconomic position, the labour process and mental health under capitalism, which generates experiences of alienation and distress across social classes (Muntaner et al, 2007).

Chapter 6

1   In view of the relatively higher costs of inpatient compared with other forms of provision (CAAPC, 2016).

2   Reference from a local newspaper (2014), withheld to preserve anonymity.

3   These figures were published in a joint Trust and local NHS Clinical Commissioning Group consultation document from 2018.

4   Reference from a local newspaper (2014), withheld to maintain the anonymity of the NHS Trust.

5   This figure was given in the Trust's 2014 Operational Plan.

[6] Roger retired in 2012; Evelyn retired in 2013; and Leslie left the RRT in 2014, three years after the SLM restructure.

[7] Steve, a social worker who had temporarily worked at Southville CMHT and been a research participant during the first phase of data collection, was also a participant in this second phase.

[8] Although cost reduction may not be the only driver of this process (it may, for instance, have progressive dimensions in so far as it heralds a greater role for peer support workers with lived experience), financial considerations are primary for Trust senior managers.

[9] A pseudonym for a high-profile private healthcare provider.

[10] The intention here is not to minimise the power inequalities between managers and workers in earlier structures of provision, but merely to suggest a contemporary shift in dominant modes of managerial control.

[11] As well as the risks associated with reductions in social and practical support, Spandler (2016) notes that there is strong evidence for the adverse and harmful physical health impacts of long-term psychotropic medication use (see Hutton et al, 2013).

[12] The Care Quality Commission (CQC) is the regulator of mental health and other care services in England.

[13] While it is the effects of more recent changes to inpatient provision that are highlighted here, longstanding concerns about the prevalence of forms of coercion and violence in this setting, including physical restraint and forcibly administered medication, should also be acknowledged (McKeown et al, 2019).

[14] While the AMHP role is now open to other professions, since Kerry (an occupational therapist) left the RRT, all the team's AMHPs were social workers.

[15] In this comment, Martin is referring to the sign that read 'Arbeit mach frei' at the entrance to the Nazi concentration camp at Auschwitz. The comparison was intended to emphasise the brutality of the UK government's coercive welfare reforms.

[16] The controversies over the walk-in closure were discussed in Chapter 2.

Chapter 7

[1] The Confederation of Health Service Employees (COHSE) trade union was formed in 1946 to represent NHS workers, merging with other public sector unions to form UNISON in 1993.

[2] This rule was changed in 1995 to enable members to take strike action.

[3] Hyde et al (2016, pp 65, 169) argue that a wider bullying culture has been established within the NHS as a result of neoliberal managerialism.

[4] This theoretical framework will be outlined in greater detail in the next chapter.

[5] Similarly, as a service user, a person's experience of oppressive services may drive them to become involved with a user-led movement. This expands their range of identities from service user (institutional role actor) to also include survivor movement activist (collective agent). Practitioners may, of course, also be (or have been) service users.

[6] This refers to interprofessional struggles to monopolise powerful institutional roles and resources (Rogers and Pilgrim, 2014).

[7] The fact that the author chose to conceal their identity is indicative of an atmosphere intolerant of dissent.

Chapter 8

[1] This conjunctive multiplicity is referred to as a laminated system (Bhaskar, 2010).

[2] This rejects the notion of the welfare state as somehow outside or external to capitalism.

[3]   Although, as the outsourcing of mental health services, and in particular the rapid growth of (particularly inpatient) private sector provision of mental healthcare to NHS patients in recent years illustrates, this is not a static situation (Moth et al, 2018).

[4]   In the *formal subsumption* of labour by capital, existing artisanal methods of production remained relatively unchanged, but by separating workers from the material 'conditions of labour' capitalists were able to extract surplus-value from their labour. Nonetheless, in spite these changes, the worker retained a degree of control over how the process of production was organised. However, this changed with the *real subsumption* of labour by capital, an outcome of the subsequent introduction of large-scale industrial production oriented around bigger units of production (for example factories). Here, a more fundamental technological and organisational transformation of the labour process, and a more complex division of labour, intensified production to increase productivity and realise greater surplus-value. This resulted in workers losing their remaining elements of independence and control over the production process (Marx, 1990).

[5]   A pentimento is an underlying image in a painting that shows through when the top layer of paint has become transparent with age. The notion developed here is indebted to, but significantly theoretically reconstructs, the account developed by Rhodes (1993).

[6]   One aspect of culture that is particularly relevant to the study of mental health services is the forms of knowledge known as the 'models of mental health'. I will propose a threefold categorisation of knowledge in the context of the mental health system, which incorporates these. This approach draws on and extends the work of Floersch (2002). 'Formal theoretical knowledge' refers to the various explanatory models, for instance biomedical or social models, that may be identified with particular mental health professions (for example, the biomedical model with psychiatry). Formal theoretical models (or 'disciplinary knowledge') constitute a basic component of the conditions for professional practice. The second type, 'applied knowledge', takes the form of local policies and formalised ways of working, shaped by team requirements and experiences, for example, locally developed assessment protocols. The third, 'contextually situated knowledge', refers to the specific, local and contingent forms of knowing produced in everyday practice and interaction between practitioners and service users, which is not mediated by formal theory (Floersch, 2002).

[7]   These cultural forms (theoretical and applied knowledge) are to be differentiated from the spontaneous ideas (contextually situated knowledge) that arise within, and thereby energise and motivate, the 'lifeworld' of human activity (Creaven, 2000).

[8]   Marx recognised this process, arguing in *The Eighteenth Brumaire of Louis Bonaparte* both that traditional institutions and practices 'inherited from the past' weigh heavily on people in the present but also that people have the collective capacities to create and recreate societies anew (Marx, 1996).

[9]   Although structures/cultures have their own autonomous causal powers, this is mediated by agential action as the only source of efficient causality, and thus an argument against reification (Archer, 1995).

[10] For a plausible general account of social interaction, a focus on rule-governed action within organisational roles is necessary but not sufficient and must be extended to include interest-governed agency related to social positions within society (at the macro level).

[11] Creaven (2000) substitutes 'collective agency' for Archer's (1995) term 'corporate agency'.

[12] In Emergentist Marxism, each interactant may be, simultaneously, an individual (primary agent), member of an organisational, occupational and/or user group (institutional role actor) and involved in political collectivities such as trade unions or social movements (collective agent). This stratified understanding of action offers analytic purchase on the ways people navigate their positional interests and engage in conflicts over power and

resources within contested organisational settings (Creaven, 2000). This theme will be developed in Chapter 9.

[13] This is in no way intended to minimise the historic and contemporary harms associated with biomedical reductionism, pharmaceuticalisation and biomedical psychiatry in mental health services, as I hope I have made clear throughout this text. However, my argument is that to reduce the harms associated with mental distress to a critique of biomedical approaches and psychiatry is to engage in a partial analysis that overlooks wider concerns about the relationship between capitalism, its institutions and lived experiences of mental distress (Sedgwick, 2015; Ferguson, 2017a).

[14] However, rather than in conflict, these market-oriented consent and punitive coercion dynamics reflect the dialectical interplay of care and control in what Gramsci characterises as the 'integral' state in its neoliberal form (Greener et al, 2019).

Chapter 9

[1] There is extensive evidence of the importance of relationships and their quality for recovery (in the grassroots sense) (Pilgrim et al, 2009; Mental Health Foundation, 2016).

[2] A particularly relevant element of this for the biomedical framework is its conceptual baggage, which includes the role of discriminatory eugenic ideas in shaping its development – see Chapter 4.

[3] Described by Sedgwick (2015) as boundary disputes 'between the fragments'.

[4] Although critical psychologists have, of course, contributed in important ways to challenging neoliberal reform through Psychologists for Social Change, and critiquing existing power inequalities in services through the Power Threat Meaning (PTM) Framework. This profession, like others, is a site of ethico-political contestation.

[5] Although, as with other mental health professions, radical and critical strands within psychiatry remain visible (Bracken and Thomas, 2005; Double, 2006).

[6] As advocated in Chapter 3 by service user Ben.

[7] 'Social justice tools' such as the Unrecovery Star enable such a focus to be visualised (Recovery in the Bin, 2019).

Conclusion

[1] This also applies to the disciplinary hierarchies that may undermine joint working between professional groups (Fulford, 2008).

[2] The example given by Harootunian (2015, p 54) is Marx's view on the communal/egalitarian political possibilities of the Russian rural communes (*obschina*) as a model for societal organisation under socialism.

[3] This critique cedes no ground to neoliberal reformers, however, as these earlier harms are counterposed to those of 'psychiatric neglect' during the current era of consumerisation and cuts (Spandler, 2016).

Appendix

[1] Formal written consent was obtained from all practitioner, service user and carer participants included in the study.

References

Abbott, P. and Wallace, C. (eds) (1990) The Sociology of the Caring Professions. London: Routledge.

Ackroyd, S. and P. Thompson (1999) Organizational Misbehaviour. London: Sage.

Ackroyd, S., Kirkpatrick, I. and Walker, R. (2007) Public management reform in the UK and its consequences for professional organization: a comparative analysis. Public Administration, 85(1): 9–26.

Adams, A., Perry, J. and Young, S. (2020) Improving the process of zoning in a community mental health team. BMJ Open Quality, 9:e000659. doi: 10.1136/ bmjoq-2019-000659.

Adams, V., Murphy, M. and Clarke, A. (2009) Anticipation: technoscience, life, affect, temporality. Subjectivity, 28(1): 246–265.

ADASS (Association of Directors of Adult Social Services) (2018) AMHPs, Mental Health Act Assessments and the Mental Health Social Care Workforce. ADASS [online]. Available from: www.adass.org.uk/national-findings-amhps-mental-health-act-assessments-the-mental-health-social-care-workforce (accessed 23 September 2020).

ADASS (2019) ADASS Budget Survey 2019: The human cost of failing to address the crisis in adult social care. ADASS [online]. Available from: https://www.adass.org.uk/adass-budget-survey-2019 (accessed 12 March 2021).

Ahmadzadeh, Y. (2021) Everyone loses when mental health research is not diverse. But how do we measure diversity? Centre for Mental Health [online]. 4 March. Available from: https://www.centreformentalhealth.org.uk/blogs/how-do-we-measure-diversity (accessed 9 March 2021).

Alaszewski, A. and Brown, P. (2016) Time, risk and health. In J.M. Chamberlain (ed) Medicine, Risk and Power. London: Routledge, pp 52–75.

American Psychiatric Association (2013) Diagnostic and Statistical Manual of Mental Disorders (5th edn). Arlington: American Psychiatric Publishing.

Anthony, W.A. (1993) Recovery from mental illness: the guiding vision of the mental health service system in the 1990s. Psychosocial Rehabilitation Journal, 16 (4): 11–23.

Archer, M. (1995) Realist Social Theory: The Morphogenetic Approach. Cambridge: Cambridge University Press.

Archer, M.S. (2014) The generative mechanism re-configuring late modernity. In M.S. Archer (ed) Late Modernity: Trajectories towards Morphogenic Society, Social Morphogenesis. Cham: Springer, pp 93–118.

Armbruster, H. (2008) Introduction: the ethics of taking sides. In H. Armbruster and A. Laerke (eds) Ethics, Politics, and Fieldwork in Anthropology. New York: Berghahn Books, pp 1–22.

Ashir, M. and Marlowe, K. (2009) Traffic lights: a practical risk management system for community early intervention in psychosis teams. Clinical Governance: An International Journal, 14(3): 226–235.

Baginsky, M. (2013) Retaining Experienced Social Workers in Children's Services: The Challenge Facing Local Authorities in England. London: King's College London.

Bailey, D. (2012) Interdisciplinary Working in Mental Health. Houndsmill: Palgrave Macmillan.

Baines, D. (2004) Caring for nothing: work organization and unwaged labour in social services. Work, Employment and Society, 18(2): 267–295.

Baldwin, M. (2009) Authoritarianism and the attack on social work. In I. Ferguson and M. Lavalette (eds) Social Work after Baby P: Issues Debates and Alternative Perspectives. Liverpool: Liverpool Hope University Press.

Ball, S. (2003) The teacher's soul and the terrors of performativity. Journal of Education Policy, 18(2): 215–228.

Barker, C. (2008) Goliath sometimes wins: a strike of community mental health workers in Manchester. In C. Barker and M. Tyldesley (eds) Proceedings: Thirteenth International Conference on Alternative Futures and Popular Protest. Manchester: Manchester Metropolitan University.

Barkhuizen, W., Cullen, A.E., Shetty, H., Pritchard, M, Stewart, R., McGuire, P. and Patel, R. (2020) Community treatment orders and associations with readmission rates and duration of psychiatric hospital admission: a controlled electronic case register study. BMJ Open, 10(3): e035121. doi: 10.1136/ bmjopen-2019-035121.

Barrett, R. (1996) The Psychiatric Team and the Social Definition of Schizophrenia. Cambridge: Cambridge University Press.

Bartlett, P. (1999) The Poor Law of Lunacy: The Administration of Pauper Lunatics in Mid-Nineteenth Century England. London: Leicester University Press.

Bartlett, W. and Harrison, L. (1993) Quasi-markets and the National Health Service reforms. In J. Le Grand and W. Bartlett (eds) Quasi-Markets and Social Policy. Basingstoke: Macmillan, pp 68–92.

Beatty, C. and Fothergill, S. (2016) The Uneven Impact of Welfare Reform: The Financial Losses to Places and People. Project Report. Sheffield: Sheffield Hallam University.

Beck, U. (1992) Risk Society. London: Sage.

Beddoe, L. and Davys, A. (2016) Challenges in Professional Supervision: Current Themes and Models for Practice. London: Jessica Kingsley Publishers.

Bensaïd, D. (2002) Marx for Our Times: Adventures and Misadventures of a Critique. London: Verso.

Beresford, P. (2009) Whose Personalisation? Think Pieces No. 47. London: Compass.

Beresford, P. (2012) Psychiatric system survivors: an emerging movement. In N. Watson, A. Roulstone and C. Thomas (eds) Routledge Handbook of Disability Studies. London: Routledge, pp 151–164.

Beresford, P. (2013) Experiential knowledge and the reconception of madness. In S. Coles, S. Keenan and B. Diamond (eds) Madness Contested: Power and Practice. Ross-on-Wye: PCCS Books, pp 181–196.

Beresford, P. (ed) (2014) Personalisation. Bristol: Policy Press.

Beresford, P. (2016) All Our Welfare: Towards Participatory Social Policy. Bristol: Policy Press.

Beresford, P. (2019) Mad studies: campaigning against the psychiatric system and welfare reform and for something better. In E. Hart, J. Greener and R. Moth (eds) Resist the Punitive State: Grassroots Struggles Across Welfare, Housing, Education and Prisons. London: Pluto Press, pp 88–107.

Beresford, P. and Carr, S. (eds) (2018) Social Policy First Hand: An International Introduction to Participatory Social Welfare. Bristol: Policy Press.

Beresford, P., Croft, S. and Adshead, L. (2008) 'We don't see her as a social worker': a service user case study of the importance of the social worker's relationship and humanity. British Journal of Social Work, 38(7): 1388–1407.

Beresford, P., Perring, R., Nettle, M. and Wallcraft, J. (2016) From Mental Illness to a Social Model of Madness and Distress. London: Shaping Our Lives.

Bevan, G. and Hood, C. (2006) What's measured is what matters: targets and gaming in the English public health care system. Public Administration, 84 (3): 517–538.

Bhaskar, R. (1998) The Possibility of Naturalism (3rd edn). Abingdon: Routledge.

Bhaskar, R. (2008a) Dialectic: The Pulse of Freedom. Abingdon: Routledge.

Bhaskar, R. (2008b) A Realist Theory of Science. London: Verso.

Bhaskar, R. (2010) Contexts of interdisciplinarity: interdisciplinarity and climate change. In R. Bhaskar, C. Frank, K.G. Høyer, P. Naess and J. Parker (eds) Interdisciplinarity and Climate Change: Transforming Knowledge and Practice for our Global Futures. London: Routledge, pp 1–24.

Bhattacharya, T. (2017) Social Reproduction Theory: Remapping Class, Recentering Oppression. London: Pluto Press.

Bhugra, D. (2008) Professionalism and psychiatry: the profession speaks. Acta Psychiatrica Scandinavia, 118: 327–329.

Bignall, T., Jeraj, S., Helsby, E. and Butt, J. (2019) Racial Disparities In Mental Health: Literature and Evidence Review. London: Race Equality Foundation.

Bister, M. (2018) The concept of chronicity in action: everyday classification practices and the shaping of mental health care. Sociology of Health and Illness, 40(1): 38–52.

BMA (British Medical Association) (2017) Breaking Down Barriers: The Challenge of Improving Mental Health Outcomes. London: British Medical Association.

Bourdieu, P. (1977) Outline of a Theory of Practice. Cambridge: Cambridge University Press.

Bracken, P. and Thomas, P. (2005) Postpsychiatry. Oxford: Oxford University Press.

Braverman, H. (1974) Labor and Monopoly Capital. New York: Monthly Review Press.

Brenner, N., Peck, J. and Theodore, N. (2010) Variegated neoliberalization: geographies, modalities, pathways. Global Networks, 10(2): 182–222.

Broadhurst, K. and Mason, C. (2014) Social work beyond the VDU: foregrounding co-presence in situated practice – why face-to-face practice matters. British Journal of Social Work, 44(3): 578–595.

Brodwin, P. (2011) Futility in the practice of community psychiatry. Medical Anthropology Quarterly, 25(2): 189–208.

Brown, B. and Baker, S. (2012) Responsible Citizens: Individuals, Health and Policy under Neoliberalism. London: Anthem Press.

Brown, B. and Manning, N. (2018) Genealogies of recovery: the framing of therapeutic ambitions. Nursing Philosophy, 19(2): e12195.

Brown, P. and Calnan, M. (2009) The risks of managing uncertainty: the limitations of governance and choice, and the potential for trust. Social Policy and Society, 9(1): 13–24.

Brown, P. and Calnan, M. (2012) Trusting on the Edge: Managing Uncertainty and Vulnerability in the Midst of Serious Mental Health Problems. Bristol: Policy Press.

Brown, P., Calnan, M., Scrivener, A. and Szmukler, G. (2009) Trust in mental health services: a neglected concept. Journal of Mental Health, 18(5): 449–458.

Burawoy, M. (1998) The extended case method. Sociological Theory, 16(1): 4–34.

Burawoy, M. (2008) II. Durable domination: Gramsci meets Bourdieu. Unpublished lecture, University of Berkeley [online]. Available from: http://burawoy.berkeley.edu/Bourdieu/Lecture 2.pdf (accessed 5 November 2021).

Burns, T. (2004) Community Mental Health Teams: A Guide to Current Practices. Oxford: Oxford University Press.

Busfield, J. (1986) Managing Madness: Changing Ideas and Practice. London: Unwin Hyman.

Butler, I. and Drakeford, M. (2003) Scandal, Social Policy and Social Welfare. Houndmills: Palgrave Macmillan.

CAAPC (Commission on Adult Acute Psychiatric Care) (2016) Old Problems, New Solutions: Improving Adult In-Patient Psychiatric Care for Adults in England. London: Department of Health.

Calnan, M. and Sandford, E. (2004) Public trust in health care: the system or the doctor? Quality and Safety in Health Care, 13(2): 92–97.

Campbell, J. and Davidson, G. (2009) Coercion in the community: a situated approach to the examination of ethical challenges for mental health social workers. Ethics and Social Welfare, 3(3): 249–263.

Cannizzo, F. (2018) The shifting rhythms of academic work. On Education: Journal for Research and Debate, 1(3): 1–4.

Carey, M. (2015) The fragmentation of social work and social care: some ramifications and a critique. British Journal of Social Work, 45(8): 2406–2422.

Carr, S. (2007) Participation, power, conflict and change: theorizing dynamics of service user participation in the social care system of England and Wales. Critical Social Policy, 27(2): 266–276.

Carrigan, M. (2018) Big data, human agency, critical realism and the future of the social sciences. CR Network webinar [online]. Available from: https://www.slideshare.net/markcarrigan/big-data-human-agency-critical-realism-and-the-future-of-the-social-sciences (accessed 16 January 2021).

Carter, B. and Stevenson, H. (2012) Teachers, workforce remodelling and the challenge to labour process analysis. Work, Employment and Society, 26(3): 481–496.

Carter, B., Stevenson, H. and Passy, R. (2010) Industrial Relations in Education: Transforming the School Workforce. London: Routledge.

Centre for Mental Health (2017) Briefing 52: Adult and Older Adult Mental Health Services 2012-2016. London: Centre for Mental Health.

Clarke, J. (2004) Dissolving the public realm? The logics and limits of neo-liberalism. Journal of Social Policy, 33(1): 27–48.

Clarke, J. and Newman, J. (1997) The Managerial State: Power, Politics and Ideology in the Remaking of Social Welfare. London: Sage.

Clarke, J., Newman, J., Smith, N., Vidler, E. and Westmarland, L. (2007) Creating Citizen-Consumers: Changing Publics and Changing Public Services. London: Sage Publications.

Clarkson, P. and Challis, D. (2002) Developing performance indicators for mental health care. Journal of Mental Health, 11(3): 281–293.

Collins, B. (2019) Payments and Contracting for Integrated Care: The False Promise of the Self-Improving Health System. London: The King's Fund

Colombo, A., Bendelow, G., Fulford, B. and Williams, S. (2003) Evaluating the influence of implicit models of mental disorder on processes of shared decision making within community-based multi-disciplinary teams. Social Science & Medicine, 56(7): 1557–1570.

Coppock, V. and Hopton, J. (2000) Critical Perspectives on Mental Health. London: Routledge.

Creaven, S. (2000) Marxism and Realism: A Materialistic Application of Realism in the Social Sciences. London: Routledge.

Creaven, S. (2002) The pulse of freedom? Bhaskar's dialectic and Marxism. Historical Materialism, 10(2): 77–141.

Creaven, S. (2007) Emergentist Marxism: Dialectical Philosophy and Social Theory. London: Routledge.

Cresswell, M. and Spandler, H. (2009) Psychopolitics: Peter Sedgwick's legacy for mental health movements. Social Theory and Health, 7(2): 129–147.

Cresswell, M. and Spandler, H. (2012) The engaged academic: academic intellectuals and the psychiatric survivor movement. Social Movement Studies: Journal of Social, Cultural and Political Protest, 11(4): 138–154.

Cresswell, M. and Spandler, H. (2016) Solidarities and tensions in mental health politics: mad studies and psychopolitics. Critical and Radical Social Work, 4(3): 357–373.

Crossley, N. (2006) Contesting Psychiatry: Social Movements in Mental Health. London: Routledge.

Culpitt, I. (1999) Social Policy and Risk. London: Sage.

Cummins, I. (2020) Using Fraser's model of 'progressive neoliberalism' to analyse deinstitutionalisation and community care. Critical and Radical Social Work, 8(1): 77–93.

Curran, D. (2016) Risk, Power and Inequality in the 21st Century. Basingstoke: Palgrave Macmillan.

Curtis, T., Dellar, R., Leslie, E. and Watson, B. (2000) Mad Pride: A Celebration of Mad Culture. Truro: Chipmunka Publishing.

Daley, A., Costa, L. and Beresford, P. (2019) Madness, Violence, and Power: A Critical Collection. Toronto: University of Toronto Press.

Darlington, R. and Upchurch, M. (2012) A reappraisal of the rank-and-file versus bureaucracy debate. Capital and Class, 36(1): 77–95.

Davidson, G., Campbell, J., Shannon, C. and Mulholland, C. (2016) Models of Mental Health. London: Palgrave Macmillan.

Davies, C.A. (2008) Reflexive Ethnography (2nd edn). London: Routledge.

Davies, D. and Bhugra, D. (2004) Models of Psychopathology. Maidenhead: Open University Press.

Davies, J. (2017) Political pills: psychopharmaceuticals and neoliberalism as mutually supporting. In J. Davies (ed) The Sedated Society: The Causes and Harms of our Psychiatric Drug Epidemic. London: Palgrave Macmillan, pp 189–225.

Deacon, B.J. (2013) The biomedical model of mental disorder: a critical analysis of its validity, utility, and effects on psychotherapy research. Clinical Psychology Review, 33(7): 846–861.

Deegan, P.E. (1988) Recovery: the lived experience of rehabilitation. Psychosocial Rehabilitation Journal, 11(4): 11–19.

Dej. E. (2016) Psychocentrism and homelessness: the pathologization/ responsibilization paradox. Studies in Social Justice, 10(1): 117–135.

DH (Department of Health) (2001) The Journey to Recovery: The Government's Vision for Mental Health Care. London: Department of Health.

DH (2003) Developing Choice, Responsiveness and Equity in Health and Social Care. London: Department of Health.

DH Payment by Results Team (2012) Mental Health Clustering Booklet 2012–13. London: Department of Health [online]. Available from: http:// www.dh.gov.uk/prod_consum_dh/groups/dh_digitalassets/@dh/@en/ documents/digitalasset/dh_132656.pdf (accessed 5 November 2021).

DHSS (Department of Health and Social Security) (1988) Report of the Committee of Inquiry into the Care and Aftercare of Miss Sharon Campbell. London: HMSO.

Dillon, J. (2011) The personal is the political. In M. Rapley, J. Moncrieff and J. Dillon (eds) De-Medicalizing Misery: Psychiatry, Psychology and the Human Condition. Basingstoke: Palgrave Macmillan, pp 141–157.

Dillon, J., Bullimore, P., Lampshire, D. and Chamberlin, J. (2013) The work of experience-based experts. In J. Read and J. Dillon (eds) Models of Madness Edition (2nd edn). Hove: Routledge, pp 305–318.

Donati, P. (2016) The 'relational subject' according to a critical realist relational sociology. Journal of Critical Realism, 15(4): 352–375.

Donati, P. and Archer, M. (2015) The Relational Subject. Cambridge: Cambridge University Press.

Double, D. (2006) Critical Psychiatry: The Limits of Madness. Basingstoke: Palgrave Macmillan.

Durcan, G. (2008) From the Inside: Experiences of Prison Mental Health Care. London: Sainsbury Centre for Mental Health.

Dwyer, P. and Wright, S. (2014) Universal Credit, ubiquitous conditionality and its implications for social citizenship. Journal of Poverty and Social Justice, 22(1): 27–35.

EHRC (Equality and Human Rights Commission) (2017) Disability Rights in the UK: UK Independent Mechanism. London: EHRC.

Engel, G. (1977) The need for a new medical model: a challenge for biomedicine. Science, 196: 129–136.

Eubanks, V. (2018) Automating Inequality: How High-Tech Tools Profile, Police and Punish the Poor. New York: St. Martin's Press.

Evans, T. (2016) Professional Discretion in Welfare Services: Beyond Street-Level Bureaucracy. London: Routledge.

Evetts, J. (1999) Professionalisation and professionalism: issues for interprofessional care. Journal of Interprofessional Care, 13(2): 119–128.

Evetts, J. (2003) The sociological analysis of professionalism: occupational change in the modern world. International Sociology, 18(2): 395–415.

Evetts, J. (2010) Organizational professionalism: changes, challenges and opportunities. Organizational Learning and Beyond Conference. Aarhus University, Copenhagen, Denmark, 20 October.

Evetts, J. (2011) A new professionalism? Challenges and opportunities. Current Sociology, 59(4): 406–422.

Ewbank, L., Thompson, J. and McKenna, H. (2017) NHS hospital bed numbers: past, present, future. The Kings Fund [online]. Available from: https://www.kingsfund.org.uk/publications/nhs-hospital-bed-numb ers (accessed 2 October 2017).

Fagan, J. (2013) Defending the NHS: the lessons of 1988. Socialist Review [online], 378. Available from: socialistreview.org.uk/378/defending-nhs-lessons-1988 (accessed 5 November 2021).

Fairbrother, P. and Poynter, G. (2001) State restructuring: managerialism, marketisation and the implications for labour. Competition & Change, 5(3): 311–333.

Featherstone, B., Gupta, A., Morris, K. and White, S. (2018) Protecting Children: A Social Model. Bristol: Policy Press.

Fenton, J. (2015) An analysis of 'ethical stress' in criminal justice social work in scotland: the place of values. British Journal of Social Work, 45(5): 1415–1432.

Fenwick, R. and Mark Tausig, M. (2007) Work and the political economy of stress: recontextualizing the study of mental health/illness in sociology. In W. Avison, J.D. McLeod and B. Pescosolido (eds) Mental Health, Social Mirror. New York: Springer, pp 143–167.

Ferguson, H. (2016) Researching social work practice close up: using ethnographic and mobile methods to understand encounters between social workers, children and families. British Journal of Social Work, 46: 153–168.

Ferguson, I. (2007) Increasing user choice or privatizing risk? The antinomies of personalization. British Journal of Social Work, 37: 387–403.

Ferguson, I. (2008) Reclaiming Social Work: Challenging Neo-Liberalism and Promoting Social Justice. London: Sage.

Ferguson, I. (2009) 'Another social work is possible!' Reclaiming the radical tradition. In V. Leskošek (ed) Theories and Methods of Social Work: Exploring Different Perspectives. Ljubljana: University of Ljubljana, pp 81–98.

Ferguson, I. (2017a) Politics of the Mind: Marxism and Mental Distress. London: Bookmarks.

Ferguson, I. (2017b) Hope over fear: social work education towards 2025. European Journal of Social Work, 20(3): 322–332.

Ferguson, I. and Woodward, R. (2009) Radical Social Work in Practice: Making a Difference. Bristol: Policy Press.

Ferguson, I., Ioakimidis, V. and Lavalette, M. (2018) Global Social Work in a Political Context: Radical Perspectives. Bristol: Policy Press.

Ferguson, I., Lavalette, M. and Mooney, G. (2002) Rethinking Welfare: A Critical Perspective. London: Sage.

Fernando, S. (2017) Institutional Racism in Psychiatry and Clinical Psychology: Race Matters in Mental Health. Basingstoke: Palgrave Macmillan.

Fistein, E., Holland, A., Clare, I. and Gunn, M. (2009) A comparison of mental health legislation from diverse Commonwealth jurisdictions. International Journal of Law and Psychiatry, 32: 147–155.

Flaherty, M. (2011) The Textures of Time: Agency and Temporal Experience. Philadelphia: Temple University Press.

Fletcher, D. and Wright, S. (2018) A hand up or a slap down? Criminalising benefit claimants in Britain via strategies of surveillance, sanctions and deterrence. Critical Social Policy, 38(2): 323–44.

Floersch, J. (2002) Meds, Money and Manners. New York: Columbia University Press.

Foot, C., Sonola. L., Maybin, J. and Naylor, C. (2012) Service Line Management: Can it Improve Quality and Efficiency? London: The King's Fund.

Foot, J. (2015) The Man Who Closed the Asylums: Franco Basaglia and the Revolution in Mental Health Care. London and New York: Verso.

Foster, N. (2005) Control, citizenship and 'risk' in mental health: perspectives from UK, USA and Australia. In S. Ramon and J. Williams (eds) Mental Health at the Crossroads: The Promise of the Psychosocial Approach. Aldershot: Ashgate, pp 25–38.

Foucault, M. (2001 [1961]) Madness and Civilisation. London: Routledge.

Frayne, D. (2019) The Work Cure: Critical Essays on Work and Wellness. Monmouth: PCCS Books.

Fricker, M. (2010) Epistemic Injustice: Power and the Ethics of Knowing. Oxford: Oxford University Press.

Friedli, L. (2009) Mental Health, Resilience and Inequalities: How Individuals and Communities are Affected. Copenhagen: World Health Organization Europe.

Friedli, L. and Stearn, R. (2015) Positive affect as coercive strategy: conditionality, activation and the role of psychology in UK government workfare programmes. Medical Humanities, 41: 40–47.

Fulford, K.W.M. (2008) Values-based practice: a new partner to evidence-based practice and a first for psychiatry? Mens Sana Monographs, 6(1): 10–21.

Garrett, P.M. (2005) Social work's 'electronic turn': notes on the deployment of information and communication technologies in social work with children and families. Critical Social Policy, 25(4): 529–554.

Garrett, P.M. (2020) Against stultifying classifications, for a 'new humanism': Frantz Fanon's contribution to social work's commitment to 'liberation'. British Journal of Social Work. doi: 10.1093/bjsw/bcaa134.

Gilburt, H. (2015) Mental Health Under Pressure. London: The King's Fund.

Gilburt, H. (2016) Trust finances raise concerns about the future of the Mental Health Taskforce recommendations. The King's Fund [online], 14 October. Available from: https://www.kingsfund.org.uk/blog/2016/10/trust-finances-mental-health-taskforce (accessed 2 June 2017).

Gilburt, H. (2018) Funding and staffing of NHS mental health providers: still waiting for parity. The King's Fund [online]. Available from: https://www.kingsfund.org.uk/publications/funding-staffing-mental-health-providers (accessed 5 January 2021).

Gilburt, H. (2020) Mental health care in the time of COVID-19. The King's Fund [online]. Available from: https://www.kingsfund.org.uk/blog/2020/07/mental-health-care-time-covid-19 (accessed 10 January 2021).

Gilliatt, S., Fenwick, J. and Alford, D. (2000) Public services and the consumer: empowerment or control? Social Policy and Administration, 34(3): 333–349.

Glasby, J. and Tew, J. (2015) Mental Health Policy and Practice (3rd edn). London: Palgrave Macmillan.

Goffman, E. (1961) Asylums. Harmondsworth: Penguin.

Gordon-Achebe, K., Hairston, D.R., Miller, S., Legha R. and Starks S. (2019) Origins of racism in American medicine and psychiatry. In M. Medlock, D. Shtasel, N.H. Trinh and D. Williams (eds) Racism and Psychiatry: Contemporary Issues and Interventions. Totowa, NJ: Humana Press, pp 3–19.

Gornall, J. (2013) DSM-5: a fatal diagnosis? British Medical Journal, 346: f3256.

Gottesman, I. (1991) Schizophrenia Genesis: The Origins of Madness. New York: W.H. Freeman.

Graby, S. (2015) Neurodiversity: bridging the gap between the disabled people's movement and the mental health system survivors' movement? In H. Spandler, J. Anderson and B. Sapey (eds) Madness, Distress and the Politics of Disablement. Bristol: Policy Press, pp 231–243.

Grant, A. and Gadsby, J. (2018) The Power Threat Meaning Framework and international mental health nurse education: a welcome revolution in human rights. Nurse Education Today, 68: 1–3.

Greener, J. and Moth, R. (2020) From shame to blame: structuring oppression through the de-legitimisation of mental 'illness' in austerity. Social Theory and Health. https://doi.org/10.1057/s41285-020-00148-8.

Greener, J., Hart, E.L. and Moth, R. (2019) Resisting the punitive state-corporate nexus: activist strategy and the integrative transitional approach. In E.L. Hart, J. Greener and R. Moth (eds) Resist the Punitive State: Grassroots Struggles across Welfare, Housing, Education and Prisons. London: Pluto Press, pp 3–27.

Gregor, C. (2010) Unconscious aspects of statutory mental health social work: emotional labour and the approved mental health professional. Journal of Social Work Practice, 24: 429–443.

Hacking, I. (2002) Mad Travelers: Reflections on the Reality of Transient Mental Illnesses. Cambridge, MA: Harvard University Press.

Hall, R. (2010) Renewing and revising the engagement between labour process theory and technology. In P. Thompson and C. Smith (eds) Working Life: Renewing Labour Process Analysis. Basingstoke: Palgrave Macmillan, pp 159–181.

Hammersley, M. and Atkinson, P. (2007) Ethnography: Principles in Practice (3rd edn). Abingdon: Routledge.

Hardin, R. (1992) The street-level epistemology of trust. Analyse and Kritik, 14(1): 152–176.

Hare Duke, L., Furtado, V., Guo, B. and Völlm, B.A. (2018) Long-stay in forensic-psychiatric care in the UK. Social Psychiatry and Psychiatric Epidemiology, 53(3): 313–321.

Harman, C. (2008) Theorising neoliberalism. International Socialism, 117: 87–121.

Harman, C. (2010) Zombie Capitalism: Global Crisis and the Relevance of Marx. Chicago: Haymarket.

Harms-Smith, L. and Nathane, M. (2018) #NotDomestication #NotIndigenisation: decoloniality in social work education. Southern African Journal of Social Work and Social Development, 30(1): 1–18.

Harootunian, H. (2015) Marx After Marx History and Time in the Expansion of Capitalism. New York: Columbia University Press.

Harper, D. and Speed, E. (2012) Uncovering recovery: the resistible rise of recovery and resilience. Studies in Social Justice , 6(1): 9–25.

Harris, J. (1998) Scientific management, bureau-professionalism, new managerialism: the labour process of state social work. British Journal of Social Work, 28(6): 839–862.

Harris, J. (1999) State social work and social citizenship in Britain: from clientelism to consumerism. British Journal of Social Work, 29(6): 915–37.

Harris J. (2003) The Social Work Business. London: Routledge.

Harris, J. (2008) State social work: constructing the present from moments in the past. British Journal of Social Work, 38 (4): 662–79.

Harris, J. (2018) T.H. Marshall is (almost) dead and buried: a response to Filipe Duarte. Critical and Radical Social Work, 6(3): 377–386.

Harris, J. and Unwin, P. (2009) Performance management in modernised social work. In J. Harris and V. White (eds) Modernising Social Work: Critical Considerations. Bristol: Policy Press pp 9–30.

Harris, J. and White, V. (eds) (2009) Modernising Social Work: Critical Considerations. Bristol: Policy Press.

Harrison, P. and Burke, B. (2020) No longer pleading for humanity. Critical and Radical Social Work, 8(3): 297–304.

Harrison, S. (2009) Co-optation, commodification and the medical model: governing UK medicine since 1991. Public Administration, 87(2): 184–197.

Harvey, D. (1989) The Condition of Postmodernity. Oxford: Blackwell.

Harvey, D. (2005) A Brief History of Neoliberalism. Oxford: Oxford University Press.

Hautamäki, L. (2018) Uncertainty work and temporality in psychiatry: how clinicians and patients experience and manage risk in practice? Health, Risk and Society, 20(1–2): 43–62.

Hayward, S. and Fee, E. (1992) More in sorrow than in anger: the British nurses' strike of 1988. International Journal of Health Services, 22(3): 397–415.

Healy, D. (2002) The Creation of Psychopharmacology. Cambridge: Harvard University Press.

Healy, D. (2006) The latest mania: selling bipolar disorder. PLoS Medicine, 3(4). Available from: http://www.plosmedicine.org/article/info:doi/10.1371/journal.pmed.0030185 (accessed 1 June 2012).

Healy, D. (2008) Mania: A Short History of Bipolar Disorder. Baltimore: Johns Hopkins University Press.

Helm, T. and Campbell, D. (2018) Number of NHS beds for mental health patients slumps by 30%. The Guardian [online]. Available from: https://www.theguardian.com/society/2018/jul/21/nhs-beds-number-mental-health-patients-falls (accessed 5 January 2021).

Henshall, C., Doherty, A., Green, H., Westcott, L. and Aveyard, H. (2018) The role of the assistant practitioner in the clinical setting: a focus group study. BMC Health Services Research, 18: 695 [online]. Available from: https://doi.org/10.1186/s12913-018-3506-y (accessed 11 November 2021).

Hewitt, J. (2008) Dangerousness and mental health policy. Journal of Psychiatric and Mental Health Nursing, 15(3): 186–194.

Hogarth, T., Hasluck, C., Pierre, G., Winterbottam, M. and Vivian, D. (2001) Work-Life Balance 2000: Results from the Baseline Study: Summary Report. Sheffield: Department for Education and Employment.

Hopton, J. (2006) The future of critical psychiatry. Critical Social Policy, 26 (1): 57–73.

Howe, D. (1996) Surface and depth in social-work practice. In N. Parton (ed) Social Theory, Social Change and Social Work. London: Routledge, pp 77–97.

Hutton, P., Weinmann, S., Bola, J. R. and Read, J. (2013) 'Antipsychotic drugs'. In J. Read and J. Dillon (eds) Models of Madness: Psychological, Social and Biological Approaches to Psychosis (2nd edn). Hove: Routledge, pp 105–124.

Hyde, P., Granter, E., Hassard, J. and McCann, L. (2016) Deconstructing the Welfare State: Managing Healthcare in the Age of Reform. London: Routledge.

Ironside, M. and Seifert, R. (2004) 'The impact of privatisation and marketisation on employment conditions in the public services'. Radical Statistics, 86: 57–71.

Jacobs, R. (2014) Payment by Results for mental health services: economic considerations of case-mix funding. Advances in Psychiatric Treatment, 20(3): 155–164.

Jeffrey, C. (2008) Guest editorial: waiting. Society and Space, 26(6): 954–958.

Jessop, B. (1999) The changing governance of welfare: recent trends in its primary functions, scale, and modes of coordination. Social Policy & Administration, 33(4): 348–359.

Jobling, H. (2014) Using ethnography to explore causality in mental health policy and practice. Qualitative Social Work, 13(1): 49–68.

Jobling, H. (2019) The legal oversight of community treatment orders: a qualitative analysis of tribunal decision-making. International Journal of Law and Psychiatry, 62: 95–103.

Johnson, S., Dalton-Locke, C., Juan, N.V.S., Foye, U., Oram, S., Papamichail, A., et al and COVID-19 Mental Health Policy Research Unit Group (2020) Impact on mental health care and on mental health service users of the COVID-19 pandemic: a mixed methods survey of UK mental health care staff. Social Psychiatry and Psychiatric Epidemiology, 56: 25–37.

Johnstone, L. and Boyle, M. with Cromby, J., Dillon, J., Harper, D., Kinderman, P. et al (2018) The Power Threat Meaning Framework. Leicester: British Psychological Society.

Johnstone, L., Boyle, M., Cromby, J. Dillon, J., Harper, D., Kinderman, P. et al (2019) Reflections on responses to the Power Threat Meaning Framework one year on. Clinical Psychology Forum, 313: 47–54.

Joint Commissioning Panel for Mental Health (2013) Guidance for Commissioners of Community Specialist Mental Health Services. London: JCPMH.

Jones, D., Visser, M., Stokes, P., Örtenblad, A., Deem, R., Rogers, P. and Tarba, S.Y. (2020) The performative university: 'targets', 'terror' and 'taking back freedom' in academia. Management Learning, 51(4): 363–377.

Jones-Berry, S. (2016) Downbanded or deleted: how the NHS is shedding its senior nurses. Nursing Standard, 30(26): 12–13.

Jordan, B. (2007) Social Work and Well-Being. Lyme Regis: Russell House.

Joyce, S. (2020) Rediscovering the cash nexus, again: subsumption and the labour–capital relation in platform work. Capital and Class, 44(4): 541–552.

Kalidindi, S., Edwards, T. and Killaspy, H. (2012) Community Psychosis Services: The Role of Community Mental Health Rehabilitation Teams. London: Royal College of Psychiatrists.

Karsten, M. (2021) Dislocated dialogue: an anthropological investigation of digitisation among professionals in fire safety. Organization, 28(1): 92–114.

Keating, F. (2007) African and Caribbean Men and Mental Health: Better Health Briefing 5. London: Race Equality Foundation.

Kemshall, H. (2002) Risk, Social Policy and Welfare. Buckingham: Open University Press.

Kemshall, H. (2011) Crime and risk: contested territory for risk theorising. International Journal of Law, Crime and Justice, 39(4): 218–229.

Kendler, K.S. (2015) A joint history of the nature of genetic variation and the nature of schizophrenia. Molecular Psychiatry, 20(1): 77–83.

Kessler, I. and Spilsbury, K. (2019) The development of the new assistant practitioner role in the English National Health Service: a critical realist perspective. Sociology of Health and Illness. doi: 10.1111/1467-9566.12983.

Kingdon, D., Solomka, B., McAllister-Williams, H., Turkington, D. Gregoire, A. et al (2012) Care clusters and mental health Payment by Results. British Journal of Psychiatry, 200(2): 162. doi: 10.1192/bjp.200.2.162.

Kirsh, B. and Tate, E. (2006) Developing a comprehensive understanding of the working alliance in community mental health. Qualitative Health Research, 16(8): 1054–1074.

Klinenburg, E. (2018) Palaces for the People: How To Build a More Equal and United Society. London: The Bodley Head.

Lacasse, J.R. and Leo, J. (2005) Serotonin and depression: a disconnect between the advertisements and the scientific literature. PLoS Med, 2(12): e392.

Laing, R.D. (1990 [1960]) The Divided Self: An Existential Study in Sanity and Madness. London: Penguin Books.

Lammi, I. (2021) Automating to control: the unexpected consequences of modern automated work delivery in practice. Organization, 28(1): 115–131.

Langan, M. (1990) Community care in the 1990s: the community care White Paper: 'Caring for People'. Critical Social Policy, 10(29): 58–70.

Laurance, J. (2003) Pure Madness: How Fear Drives the Mental Health System. London: Routledge.

Lavalette, M. (2007) Social work: a profession worth fighting for? In G. Mooney and A. Law (eds) New Labour/Hard Labour: Restructuring and Resistance Inside The Welfare Industry. Bristol: Policy Press, pp 189–208.

Lavalette, M. and Penketh, L. (2003) The welfare state in the United Kingdom. In C. Aspalter (ed) Welfare Capitalism Around the World. Hong Kong: Casa Verde Publishing, pp 61–86.

Law, A. and Mooney, G. (2007) Strenuous welfarism: restructuring the welfare labour process. In G. Mooney and A. Law (eds) New Labour/ Hard Labour? Restructuring and Resistance Within the Welfare Industry. Bristol: Policy Press, pp 23–52.

Layard, R. (2005) Happiness: Lessons from a New Science. London: Penguin.

Layder, D. (1993) Strategies in Social Research: An Introduction and Guide. Cambridge: Polity Press.

Layder, D. (1997) Modern Social Theory: Key Debates and New Directions. London: UCL Press.

Layder, D. (1998) Sociological Practice: Linking Theory and Research. London: Sage.

Le Francois, B., Menzies, R. and Reaume, G. (eds) (2013) Mad Matters: A Critical Reader In Canadian Mad Studies. Toronto: Canadian Scholars Press.

Leader, D. (2012) What is Madness? London: Penguin.

Learmonth, M. (2005) Doing things with words: the case of 'management' and 'administration'. Public Administration, 83(3): 617–637.

Lee, C., Hartley, C. and Sharland, E. (2017) Risk thinking and the priorities of mental health social work organisations. In S. Stanford, E. Sharland, N.R. Heller and J. Warner (eds) Beyond the Risk Paradigm in Mental Health Policy and Practice. London: Palgrave, pp 30–44.

Lester, H. and Glasby, J. (2010) Mental Health Policy and Practice (2nd edn). Houndmills: Palgrave Macmillan.

Lethbridge, J. (2019) Democratic Professionalism in Public Services. Bristol: Policy Press.

Lilo, E. and Vose, C. (2016) Mental Health Integration Past, Present and Future: Report of National Survey into Mental Health Integration in England. Liverpool: Merseycare Foundation Trust/Health Education North West.

Lindisfarne, N. (2008) Starting from below: fieldwork, gender and imperialism now. In H. Armbruster and A. Laerke (eds) Ethics, Politics, and Fieldwork in Anthropology. New York: Berghahn Books, pp 23–44.

Link, B. and Phelan, J. (1999) The labeling theory of mental disorder (ii): the consequences of labeling. In A.V. Horwitz and T.L. Scheid (eds) A Handbook for the Study of Mental Health. Cambridge: Cambridge University Press, pp 361–376.

Lister, J. (2008) The NHS after 60: For Patients or Profits? London: Middlesex University Press.

Luhrmann, T. (2001) Of Two Minds: An Anthropologist Looks at American Psychiatry. New York: Vintage Books.

Mad Covid (no date) Mad Covid [online]. Available from: https://madco vid.wordpress.com/ (accessed 10 February 2021).

Maielli, G. (2015) Explaining organizational paths through the concept of hegemony: evidence from the Italian car industry. Organization Studies, 36(4): 491–511.

Marx, K. (1990 [1867]) Capital: A Critique of Political Economy, Vol 1. Harmondsworth: Penguin.

Marx, K. (1993 [1861]) Grundrisse: Foundations of the Critique of Political Economy. London: Penguin.

Marx, K. (1996 [1852]) The eighteenth brumaire of Louis Bonaparte. In K. Marx, and T. Carver (eds) Later Political Writings. Cambridge: Cambridge University Press, pp 31–127

Mather, K. and Seifert, R. (2017) Heading for disaster: extreme work and skill mix changes in the emergency services of England. Capital & Class, 41(1): 3–22.

Mathers, A., Upchurch, M. and Taylor, G. (2018) Social movement theory and trade union organizing. In J. Grote and C. Wagemann (eds) Social Movements and Organized Labour: Passions and Interests. Aldershot: Ashgate.

McDonald, C. (2006) Challenging Social Work: The Context of Practice. Basingstoke: Palgrave Macmillan.

McKenzie, K., Samele, C., Van Horn, E., Tattan, T., Van Os, J. and Murray, R. (2001) Comparison of the outcome and treatment of psychosis in people of Caribbean origin living in the UK and British Whites: report from the UK700 trial. British Journal of Psychiatry, 178(2): 160–165.

McKenna, D., Peters, P. and Moth, R. (2019) Resisting the work cure: mental health, welfare reform and the movement against psychocompulsion. In M. Berghs, T. Chataika, Y. El-Lahib and K. Dube (eds) The Routledge Handbook of Disability Activism. London: Routledge, pp 128–153.

McKeown, M. (2009) Alliances in action: opportunities and threats to solidarity between workers and service users in health and social care disputes. Social Theory and Health, 7(2): 148–169.

McKeown, M. (2020) Love and resistance: re-inventing radical nurses in everyday struggles. Journal of Clinical Nursing, 29(7–8): 1023–1025.

McKeown, M., Cresswell, M. and Spandler, H. (2014) Deeply engaged relationships: alliances between mental health workers and psychiatric survivors in the UK. In Psychiatry Disrupted: Theorizing Resistance and Crafting the (R)evolution. Montreal: McGill/Queen's University Press, pp 145–162.

McKeown, M., Scholes, A., Jones, F. and Aindow, W. (2019) Coercive practices in mental health services: stories of recalcitrance, resistance, and legitimation. In A. Daley, L. Costa and P. Beresford (eds) Madness, Violence, and Power. Toronto: University of Toronto Press, pp 263–285.

McNally, D. (2015) The dialectics of unity and difference in the constitution of wage- labour: on internal relations and working-class formation. Capital & Class, 39(1): 131–146.

McWade, B. (2015) Temporalities of mental health recovery. Subjectivity, 8(3): 243–260.

McWade, B. (2016) Recovery-as-policy as a form of neoliberal state making. Intersectionalities: A Global Journal of Social Work Analysis, Research, Polity and Practice, 5(3): 62–81.

Mental Health Foundation (2016) Relationships in the 21st Century: The Forgotten Foundation of Mental Health and Wellbeing. London: Mental Health Foundation.

Mental Health Taskforce (2016) The Five Year Forward View for Mental Health. London: NHS England.

Mills, C. (2014) Decolonizing Global Mental Health: The Psychiatrization of the Majority World. London: Routledge.

Miresco, M.J. and Kirmayer, L. J. (2006) The persistence of mind-brain dualism in psychiatric reasoning about clinical scenarios. American Journal of Psychiatry, 163(5): 913–918.

Moncrieff, J. (2008) Neoliberalism and biopsychiatry: a marriage of convenience. In C.I. Cohen and S. Timimi (eds) Liberatory Psychiatry: Philosophy, Politics and Mental Health. Cambridge: Cambridge University Press, pp 235–256.

Monitor (2006) How Service-Line Reporting Can Improve the Productivity and Performance of NHS Foundation Trusts. London: Monitor.

Moore, P. (2018) The Quantified Self in Precarity: Work, Technology and What Counts. London: Routledge.

Moore, P.V., Akhtar, P. and Upchurch, M. (2018) Digitalisation of work and resistance. In P.V. Moore, M. Upchurch and X. Whittaker (eds) Humans and Machines at Work. Basingstoke: Palgrave Macmillan, pp 17–44.

Moth, R. (2014) 'The business end': perspectives on mental distress in the context of neoliberal restructuring of community mental health services. Unpublished PhD Thesis, University of Birmingham.

Moth, R. (2020) 'The business end': neoliberal policy reforms and biomedical residualism in frontline community mental health practice in England. Competition and Change, 24(2): 133–153.

Moth, R. (forthcoming a) Sedimented structures and situational logics in England's mental health system: theorising perspectives on mental distress in socio-historical context. Journal of Critical Realism.

Moth, R. (forthcoming b) Traps, gaps and benefits distress: theorising the social and psychological harms of welfare reform for claimants with mental health needs. Article in preparation.

Moth, R. and Lavalette, M. (2017) Social Protection and Labour Market Policies for Vulnerable Groups from a Social Investment Perspective: The Case of Welfare Recipients with Mental Health Needs in England. Liverpool: Liverpool Hope University/Leuven: HIVA (KU Leuven).

Moth, R. and Lavalette, M. (2019) Social policy and welfare movements 'from below': the Social Work Action Network (SWAN) in the UK. In U. Klammer, S. Leiber and S. Leitner (eds) Social Work and the Making of Social Policy. Bristol: Policy Press, pp 121–136.

Moth, R. and McKeown, M. (2016) Realising Sedgwick's vision: theorising strategies of resistance to neoliberal mental health and welfare policy. Critical and Radical Social Work, 4(3): 375–390.

Moth, R., Greener, J. and Stoll, T. (2015) Crisis and resistance in mental health services in England. Critical and Radical Social Work, 3(1): 89–101.

Moth, R., Neary, D. and Lavalette, M. in collaboration with Baeten, R., Elsinga, M.G., Haffner, M., et al (2018) Towards Inclusive Service Delivery through Social Investment in England. An Analysis of Five Sectors, with a Particular Focus on Mental Health. Liverpool: Liverpool Hope University/Leuven: HIVA.

Muijen, M. (1996) Scare in the community: Britain in moral panic. In T. Heller, J. Reynolds, R. Gomm, R. Muston and S. Pattison (eds) Mental Health Matters. Houndmills: Palgrave Macmillan, pp 143–156.

Muntaner, C. and Geiger-Brown, J. (2006) Mental health. In B.S. Levy and V.W. Sidel (eds) Social Injustice and Public Health. Oxford: Oxford University Press, pp 277–293.

Muntaner, C., Borrell, C. and Chung, H. (2007) Class relations, economic inequality and mental health: why social class matters to the sociology of mental health. In W. Avison, J.D. McLeod and B. Pescosolido (eds) Mental Health, Social Mirror. New York: Springer, pp 127–141.

Mutch, A. (2019) Reframing Institutional Logics: History, Substance and Practices. London: Routledge.

Mutch, A. (2020) Margaret Archer and a morphogenetic take on strategy. Critical Perspectives on Accounting, 73. doi: 10.1016/j.cpa.2016.06.007.

National Audit Office (2018) Financial Sustainability of Local Authorities 2018. London: National Audit Office.

Nazroo, J.Y., Bhui, K.S. and Rhodes, J. (2020) Where next for understanding race/ethnic inequalities in severe mental illness? Structural, interpersonal and institutional racism. Sociology of Health & Illness, 42(2): 262–276.

Newbigging, K. and Ridley, J. (2018) Epistemic struggles: the role of advocacy in promoting epistemic justice and rights in mental health. Social Science & Medicine, 219: 36–44.

Newman, J. (2007) Rethinking 'the public' in troubled times: unsettling nation, state and the liberal public sphere. Public Policy and Administration, 22(1): 27–47.

NHS Benchmarking Network (2016) NHS Benchmarking Network Inpatient and Community Mental Health. November 2016. Manchester: NHS Benchmarking Network.

NHS Digital (2021) Detentions under the Mental Health Act [online]. Available from: https://www.ethnicity-facts-figures.service.gov.uk/health/mental-health/detentions-under-the-mental-health-act/latest (accessed 30 July 2021).

NHS Improvement (2019) 2019/20 National Tariff Payment System – A Consultation Notice: Annex DtE Technical Guidance for Mental Health Clusters. London: NHS Improvement.

Norman, I. and Peck, E. (1999) Working together in adult community mental health teams: an inter-professional dialogue. Journal of Mental Health, 8(3): 217–30.

Nutt, K. and Keville, S. (2016) '… you kind of frantically go from one thing to the next and there isn't any time for thinking any more': a reflection on the impact of organisational change on relatedness in multidisciplinary teams. Reflective Practice, 17(2): 221–232.

O'Brien, M. (2000) Class struggle and the English Poor Laws. In M. Lavalette and G. Mooney (eds) Class Struggle and Social Welfare. London: Routledge, pp 13–33.

O'Donnell, A. and Shaw, M. (2016) Resilience and resistance on the road to recovery in mental health. The Journal of Contemporary Community Education Practice Theory, 7(3): 1–18.

O'Leary, P., Tsui, M. and Ruch, G. (2013) The boundaries of the social work relationship revisited: towards a connected, inclusive and dynamic conceptualization. British Journal of Social Work, 43(1): 135–153.

O'Neill, L. (2015) Regulating hospital social workers and nurses: propping up an "efficient" lean health care system. Studies in Political Economy, 95(1): 115–136.

Olende, K. (2020) The hostile environment for immigrants, the Windrush scandal and resistance. In E.L. Hart, J. Greener and R. Moth (eds) Resist the Punitive State: Grassroots Struggles across Welfare, Housing, Education and Prisons. London: Pluto Press, pp 149–170.

Onyett, S. (2003) Teamworking in Mental Health. Houndmills: Palgrave Macmillan.

Onyett, S., Pillinger, T. and Muijen, M. (1997) Job satisfaction and burnout among members of community mental health teams. Journal of Mental Health, 6(1): 55–66.

Parker, I., Georgaca, E., Harper, D., McLaughlin, T. and Stowell-Smith, M. (1995) Deconstructing Psychopathology. London: Sage.

Parton, N. (2008) Changes in the form of knowledge in social work: from the 'social' to the 'informational'? The British Journal of Social Work, 38(2): 253–269.

Pass, J. (2018) Gramsci meets emergentist materialism: towards a neo neo-Gramscian perspective on world order. Review of International Studies, 44(4): 595–618.

Patrick, R. (2017) For Whose Benefit? The Everyday Realities of Welfare Reform. Bristol: Policy Press.

Peck, J. and Theodore, N. (2012) Reanimating neoliberalism: process geographies of neoliberalization. Social Anthropology, 20(2): 177–185.

Percy, E. (1957) Report of the Royal Commission on the Law Relating to Mental Illness and Mental Deficiency. London: HMSO.

Pfeffer, J. and Stein, G. (1998) Diagnosis, classification and measurement. In G. Stein and G. Wilkinson (eds) Seminars in General Adult Psychiatry. London: Gaskell, pp 1229–1273.

Pickersgill, M. (2019) Digitising psychiatry? Sociotechnical expectations, performative nominalism and biomedical virtue in (digital) psychiatric praxis. Sociology of Health and Illness, 41(S1): 16–30.

Pilgrim, D. (1997) Psychotherapy and Society. London: Sage.

Pilgrim, D. (2002) The biopsychosocial model in Anglo-American psychiatry: past, present and future. Journal of Mental Health, 11(6): 585–594.

Pilgrim, D. (2007) New 'mental health' legislation for England and Wales: some aspects of consensus and conflict. Journal of Social Policy, 36 (1): 79–95.

Pilgrim, D. (2008) The eugenic legacy in psychology and psychiatry. International Journal of Social Psychiatry, 54(3): 272–284.

Pilgrim, D. (2015) Understanding Mental Health: A Critical Realist Exploration. London: Routledge.

Pilgrim, D. and McCranie, A. (2013) Recovery and Mental Health: A Critical Sociological Account. Basingstoke: Palgrave Macmillan.

Pilgrim, D. and Rogers, A. (1999) Mental health policy and the politics of mental health: a three tier analytical framework. Policy & Politics, 27(1): 13–24.

Pilgrim, D. and Rogers, A. (2003) Mental disorder and violence: an empirical picture in context. Journal of Mental Health, 12(1): 7–18.

Pilgrim, D. Kinderman, P. and Tai, S. (2008) Taking stock of the biopsychosocial model in the field of 'mental health care'. Journal of Social and Psychological Sciences, 1(2): 1–39.

Pilgrim, D., Rogers, A. and Bentall, R. (2009) The centrality of personal relationships in the creation and amelioration of mental health problems: the current interdisciplinary case. Health: An Interdisciplinary Journal for the Social Study of Health, Illness and Medicine, 13(2): 235–254.

Pilgrim, D., Tomasini, F. and Vassilev, I. (2011) Examining Trust in Healthcare: A Multidisciplinary Perspective. Basingstoke: Palgrave Macmillan.

Pithouse, A., Broadhurst, K., Hall, C., Peckover, S., Wastell, D. and White, S. (2012) Trust, risk and the (mis)management of contingency and discretion through new information technologies in children's services. Journal of Social Work, 12(2): 158–178.

Platt, L. and Warwick, R. (2020) Are Some Ethnic Groups More Vulnerable to COVID-19 than Others? London: Institute for Fiscal Studies and Nuffield Foundation.

Polanyi, M. (1958) Personal Knowledge: Towards a Post-Critical Philosophy. Chicago: University of Chicago Press.

Pollock, A. and Price, D. (2011) The final frontier: the UK's new coalition government turns the English National Health Service over to the global health care market. Health Sociology Review, 20(3): 294–305.

Pollock, A., Price, D., Talbot-Smith, A. and Mohan, J. (2003) The NHS and the Health and Social Care Bill: end of Bevan's vision? British Medical Journal, 327: 982–985.

Porter, R. (1987) Mind-Forg'd Manacles: A History of Madness in England from the Restoration to the Regency. London: Athlone Press.

Pritchard, C. (2006) Mental Health Social Work. Houndmills: Palgrave Macmillan.

Raco, M. (2009) From expectations to aspirations: state modernisation, urban policy, and the existential politics of welfare in the UK. Political Geography, 28(7): 436–444.

Ramon, S. (2005) Approaches to risk in mental health: a multidisciplinary discourse. In J. Tew (ed) Social Perspectives in Mental Health: Developing Social Models to Understand and Work with Mental Distress. London: Jessica Kingsley Publishers, pp 184–199.

Ramon, S. (2006) British mental health social work and the psychosocial approach in context. In D. Double (ed) Critical Psychiatry: The Limits of Madness. Basingstoke: Palgrave Macmillan, pp 133–148.

Ramon, S. (2007) Inequality in mental health: the relevance of current research and understanding to potentially effective social work responses. Radical Psychology, 6(1) [online]. Available from: http://www.radpsynet.org/journal/vol6-1/ramon.htm (accessed 8 September 2012).

Ramon, S. (2008) Neoliberalism and its implications for mental health in the UK. International Journal of Law and Psychiatry, 31: 116–125.

Ramon, S., Healy, B. and Renouf, N. (2007) Recovery from mental illness as an emergent concept and practice in Australia and the UK. International Journal of Social Psychiatry, 53(2): 108–122.

Ravalier, J.M. (2019) Psycho-social working conditions and stress in UK social workers. The British Journal of Social Work, 49(2): 371–390.

Read, J. and Bentall, R. (2012) Negative childhood experiences and mental health. The British Journal of Psychiatry, 200(2): 89–91.

Read, J. and Dillon, J. (eds) (2013) Models of Madness: Psychological, Social and Biological Approaches to Schizophrenia (2nd edn). Hove: Brunner-Routledge.

Recovery in the Bin (2019) Unrecovery. In D. Frayne (ed) The Work Cure: Critical Essays on Work and Wellness. Monmouth: PCCS Books, pp 227–249.

Recovery in the Bin, Edwards, B.M., Burgess, R. and Thomas, E. (2019) Neorecovery: a survivor led conceptualisation and critique [transcript]. Keynote presented at the 25th International Mental Health Nursing Research Conference, The Royal College of Nursing, London, UK. Available from: https://recoveryinthebin.org/2019/09/16/__trashed-2/ (accessed 5 November 2021).

Reid, A. (2003) Understanding teachers' work: is there still a place for labour process theory? British Journal of Sociology of Education, 24(5): 559–573.

Repper, J. (2013) Peer Support Workers: Theory and Practice. London: Centre for Mental Health.

Repper, J. and Perkins, R. (2003) Social Inclusion and Recovery. Edinburgh: Bailliere Tindall.

Rhodes, L. (1993) The shape of action: practice in public psychiatry. In S. Lindenbaum and L. Lock (eds) Knowledge Power and Practice: The Anthropology of Medicine and Everyday Life. Berkeley, CA: University of California Press, pp 129–144.

Ridley, J. and Jones, L. (2003) Direct what? The untapped potential of direct payments to mental health service users. Disability & Society, 18(5): 643–658.

Rimke, H. (2010) Consuming fears: neoliberal in/securities, cannibalization, and psychopolitics. In J. Shantz (ed) Racism and Borders: Representation, Repression, Resistance. New York: Algora Publishing, pp 95–112.

Rimke, H. and Brock, D. (2012) The culture of therapy: psychocentrism in everyday life. In M. Thomas, R. Raby and D. Brock (eds) Power and Everyday Practices. Toronto: Nelson, pp 182–202.

Ritchie, J., Dick, D. and Lingham, R. (1994) The Report of the Inquiry into the Care and Treatment of Christopher Clunis. London: HMSO.

Robcis, C. (2016) Francois Tosquelles and the psychiatric revolution in postwar France. Constellations, 23(2): 212–223.

Roberts, G. and Wolfson, P. (2004) The rediscovery of recovery: open to all. Advances in Psychiatric Treatment, 10: 37–49.

Rogers, A. and Pilgrim, D. (2001) Mental Health Policy in Britain (2nd edn). Houndmills: Palgrave Macmillan.

Rogers, A. and Pilgrim, D. (2014) A Sociology of Mental Health and Illness (5th edn). Maidenhead: Open University Press.

Rogers, A., Bury, M. and Kennedy, A. (2009) Rationality, rhetoric, and religiosity in health care: the case of England's expert patients programme. International Journal of Health Services, 39(4): 725–747.

Roland, M. and Guthrie, B. (2016) Quality and Outcomes Framework: what have we learnt? British Medical Journal, 354: i4060.

Rosa, H. (2017) De-Synchronization, dynamic stabilization, dispositional squeeze: the problem of temporal mismatch. In J. Wajcman and N. Dodd (eds) The Sociology of Speed: Digital, Organizational, and Social Temporalities. Oxford: Oxford University Press, pp 25–41.

Rose, N. (1998a) Living dangerously: risk-thinking and risk management in mental health care. Mental Health Care, 1(8): 263–266.

Rose, N. (1998b) Governing risky individuals: the role of psychiatry in new regimes of control. Psychiatry, Psychology and Law, 5(2): 177–195.

Rosen, G. (1978) Madness in Society. New York: Harper.

Roulstone, A. (2015) Personal Independence Payments, welfare reform and the shrinking disability category. Disability & Society, 30(5): 673–688.

Roulstone, A. and Morgan, H. (2009) Neo-liberal individualism or self-directed support: are we all speaking the same language on modernising adult social care? Social Policy and Society, 8(3): 333–345.

Rugkåsa, J. and Dawson, J. (2013) Community treatment orders: current evidence and the implications. British Journal of Psychiatry, 203(6): 406–408.

Russo, J. and Beresford, P. (2015) Between exclusion and colonisation: seeking a place for mad people's knowledge in academia. Disability and Society, 30(1): 153–157.

Ryle, G. (1949) The Concept of Mind. Chicago: University of Chicago Press.

Ryrie, I., Hellard, L., Kearns, C., Robinson, D., Pathmanathan, I. and O'Sullivan, D. (1997) Zoning: a system for managing case work and targeting resources in community. Journal of Mental Health, 6(5): 515–523.

Sapey, B., Spandler, H. and Anderson, J. (2015) Introduction. In H. Spandler, J. Anderson and B. Sapey (eds) Madness, Distress and the Politics of Disablement. Bristol: Policy Press, pp 1–9.

Sass, L. (2017) Madness and Modernism: Insanity in the Light of Modern Art, Literature, and Thought (2nd edn). Oxford: Oxford University Press.

Sayer, A. (1992) Method in Social Science: A Realist Approach (2nd edn). London: Routledge.

Sayer, A. (2011) Why Things Matter to People: Social Science, Values and Ethical Life. Cambridge: Cambridge University Press.

Sayer, A. (2012) Power, causality and normativity: a critical realist critique of Foucault. Journal of Political Power, 5(2): 179–194.

Scheff, T. (1984) Being Mentally Ill: A Sociological Theory (2nd edn). New York: Aldine.

Scheherazade (2018) Power Threat Meaning Threat Power Power Power. Available from: https://recoveryinthebin.org/2018/01/16/power-threat-meaning-threat-power-power-power-review-by-scheherazade/ (accessed 1 August 2021).

Scheper-Hughes, N. (1995) The primacy of the ethical: propositions for a militant anthropology. Current Anthropology, 36(3): 409–440.

Scull, A. (1977) Madness and segregative control: the rise of the insane asylum. Social Problems, 24(3): 337–351.

Sedgwick, P. (2015 [1982]) *Psycho Politics*. London: Unkant Publishers.

Shah, A. (2018) Nightmarch: Among India's Revolutionary Guerrillas. Chicago: University of Chicago Press.

Shakespeare, T., Watson, N. and Alghaib, O. (2017) Blaming the victim, all over again: Waddell and Aylward's biopsychosocial (BPS) model of disability. Critical Social Policy, 37(1): 22–41.

Sheaff, R. and Pilgrim, D. (2006) Can learning organizations survive in the newer NHS? Implementation Science, 1(27): 1–11.

Slade, M. (2009) Personal Recovery and Mental Illness. Cambridge: Cambridge University Press.

Slasberg, C., Beresford, P. and Schofield, P. (2012) How self-directed support is failing to deliver personal budgets and personalisation. Research, Policy and Planning, 29(3): 161–177.

Smail, D. (2005) Power, Interest and Psychology: Elements of a Social Materialist Understanding of Distress. Ross-on-Wye: PCCS Books.

Smith, P. (1995) On the unintended consequences of publishing performance data in the public sector. International Journal of Public Administration, 18(2–3): 277–310.

Soldatic, K. (2013) Appointment time: disability and neoliberal workfare temporalities. Critical Sociology, 39(3): 405–419.

Spandler, H. (2004) Friend or foe: towards a critical assessment of direct payments. Critical Social Policy, 24(2): 187–209.

Spandler, H. (2006) Asylum to Action: Paddington Day Hospital, Therapeutic Communities and Beyond. London: Jessica Kingsley Publishers.

Spandler, H. (2007) From social exclusion to inclusion? A critique of the inclusion imperative in mental health. Medical Sociology Online, 2(2): 3–16.

Spandler H. (2016) From psychiatric abuse to psychiatric neglect? Asylum, 23(2): 7–8.

Spandler, H. and McKeown, M. (2017) Exploring the case for truth and reconciliation in mental health services. Mental Health Review Journal, 22(2): 83–94.

Spandler, H. and Stickley, T. (2011) No hope without compassion: the importance of compassion in recovery-focused mental health services. Journal of Mental Health, 20(6): 555–566.

Stanford, S., Heller, N., Sharland, E. and Warner, J. (2017) Moving beyond neoliberal rationalities of risk in mental health policy and practice. In S. Stanford, E. Sharland, N.R. Heller and J. Warner (eds) Beyond the Risk Paradigm in Mental Health Policy and Practice. London: Palgrave, pp 45–58.

Stanley, N. and Manthorpe, J. (2001) Reading mental health inquiries: messages for social work. Journal of Social Work, 1(1): 77–99.

Stewart, M., Brown, J., Weston, W., McWhinney, I., McWilliam, C. and Freeman, T. (2014) Patient-Centered Medicine: Transforming the Clinical Method. London: CRC Press.

Stoye, G. (2017) UK Health Spending IFS Briefing Note BN201. London: Institute for Fiscal Studies.

Sullivan, O. and Gershuny, J. (2018) Speed-up society? Evidence from the UK 2000 and 2015 Time Use Diary Surveys. Sociology, 52(1): 20–38.

Survivors History Group (2011) Survivors History Group takes a critical look at historians. In M. Barnes and P. Cotterell (eds) Critical Perspectives on User Involvement. Bristol: Policy Press, pp 7–18.

Szmukler, G. and Rose, N. (2013) Risk assessment in mental health care: values and costs. Behavioral Sciences and the Law, 31: 125–140.

Taggart, D., Rouf, K., Hisham, I., Duckworth L. and Sweeney, A. (2021) Trauma, mental health and the COVID-19 crisis: are we really all in it together? Journal of Mental Health. doi: 10.1080/09638237.2021.1875415.

Taylor, P. and Gunn, J. (1999) Homicides by people with mental illness: myth and reality. British Journal of Psychiatry, 174: 9–14.

Taylor-Gooby, P. (2016) The divisive welfare state. Social Policy & Administration, 50(6): 712–733.

Tew, J. (ed) (2005) Social Perspectives in Mental Health: Developing Social Models to Understand and Work with Mental Distress. London: Jessica Kingsley Publishers.

Tew, J. (2011) Social Approaches to Mental Distress. Houndmills: Palgrave Macmillan.

Theodore, N. (2019) Governing through austerity: (il)logics of neoliberal urbanism after the global financial crisis. Journal of Urban Affairs. doi: 10.1080/07352166.2019.1623683.

Thomas, P. (2009) The Gramscian Moment: Philosophy, Hegemony and Marxism. Leiden: Brill.

Thompson, E.P. (1967) Time, work-discipline, and industrial capitalism, Past and Present, 38(1): 56–97.

Thompson, P. and Vincent, S. (2010) Labour process theory and critical realism. In P. Thompson and C. Smith (eds) Working Life: Renewing Labour Process Analysis. Basingstoke: Palgrave Macmillan, pp 47–69.

Tickell, A. and Peck, J. (2003) Making global rules: globalization or neoliberalisation. In J. Peck and H. Yeung (eds) Remaking the Global Economy: Economic-Geographical Perspectives. London: Sage, pp 163–182.

Tomba, M. (2013) Marx's Temporalities. Leiden: Brill.

Tomba, M. (2015) Marx's temporal bridges and other pathways. Historical Materialism, 23(4): 75–91.

Toone, B., Murray, R., Clare, A., Creed, F. and Smith, A. (1979) Psychiatrists' models of mental illness and their personal backgrounds. Psychological Medicine, 9(1): 165–178.

Trevithick, L., Painter, J. and Keown, P. (2015) Mental health clustering and diagnosis in psychiatric in-patients. BJPsych Bulletin, 39(3): 119–123.

Trewin, M. (2017) Social Care and the Mental Health Forward View: Ending Out of Area Placements. London: Centre for Mental Health.

Trittin-Ulbrich, H., Scherer, A., Munro, I. and Whelan, G. (2021) Exploring the dark and unexpected sides of digitalization: toward a critical agenda. Organization, 28(1): 8–25.

Twomey, C.D., Baldwin, D.S., Hopfe, M. and Cieza, A. (2015) A systematic review of the predictors of health service utilisation by adults with mental disorders in the UK. BMJ Open, 5: e007575. doi: 10.1136/bmjopen-2015-007575.

Tyrer, P. (2013) Models for Mental Disorder: Conceptual Models in Psychiatry (5th edn). Chichester: John Wiley.

Umney, C. (2018) Class Matters: Inequality and Exploitation in 21st Century Britain. London: Pluto Press.

UN Special Rapporteur on the Right to Health (2017) Report of the Special Rapporteur on the Right of Everyone to the Enjoyment of the Highest Attainable Standard of Physical and Mental Health. New York: Office of the United Nations High Commissioner for Human Rights.

Valenstein, E. (1998) Blaming the Brain: The Truth about Drugs and Mental Health. New York: Free Press.

Valsraj, K.M. and Gardner, N. (2007) Choice in mental health: myths and possibilities. Advances in Psychiatric Treatment, 13: 60–67.

Van Os, J., Guloksuz, S., Vijn, T.W., Hafkenscheid, A. and Delespaul, P. (2019) The evidence-based group-level symptom-reduction model as the organizing principle for mental health care: time for change? World Psychiatry, 18(1): 88–96.

Von Peter, S. (2010) The temporality of 'chronic' mental illness. Culture Medicine Psychiatry, 34(1): 13–28.

Vostal, F., Benda, L. and Vortová, T. (2019) Against reductionism: on the complexity of scientific temporality. Time and Society, 28(2): 783–803.

Wajcman, J. (2008) Life in the fast lane? Towards a sociology of technology and time. British Journal of Sociology, 59(1): 59–77.

Wajcman, J. (2015) Pressed for Time: The Acceleration of Life in Digital Capitalism. Chicago: University of Chicago Press.

Wall, O. (2018) The British Anti-Psychiatrists: From Institutional Psychiatry to the Counter-Culture, 1960–1971. Abingdon: Routledge.

Wallace, S., Nazroo, J. and Becares, L. (2016) Cumulative effect of racial discrimination on the mental health of ethnic minorities in the United Kingdom. American Journal of Public Health, 106: 1294–1300.

Warner, J. (2006) Inquiry reports as active texts and their function in relation to professional practice in mental health. Health, Risk & Society, 8(3): 223–237.

Warner, J., Heller, N., Sharland, E. and Stanford, S. (2017) The historical context of the risk paradigm in mental health policy and practice: how did we get here? In S. Stanford, E. Sharland, N.R. Heller and J. Warner (eds) Beyond the Risk Paradigm in Mental Health Policy and Practice. London: Palgrave Macmillan, pp 1–16.

Warner, J., Talbot, D. and Bennison, G. (2013) The cafe as affective community space: reconceptualizing care and emotional labour in everyday life. Critical Social Policy, 33(2): 305–324.

Watkins, J., Wulaningsih, W., Da Zhou, C., Marshall, D.C., Sylianteng, G.D.C., Dela Rosa, P.G., et al (2017) Effects of health and social care spending constraints on mortality in England: a time trend analysis. BMJ Open, 7: e017722. doi: 10.1136/ bmjopen-2017-017722.

Watts, B. and Fitzpatrick, S. (2018) Welfare Conditionality. Abingdon: Routledge.

Watts, G. (2012) Critics attack DSM-5 for overmedicalising normal human behaviour. British Medical Journal, 344: e1020.

Webb, S. (2006) Social Work in a Risk Society: Social and Political Perspectives. Houndmills: Palgrave Macmillan.

Weich, S., Duncan, C., Bhui, K., Canaway, A., Crepaz-Keay, D., Keown, P., et al (2018) Evaluating the effects of community treatment orders (CTOs) in England using the Mental Health Services Dataset (MHSDS): protocol for a national, population-based study. BMJ Open, 8: e024193.

White, M. (1997) Narratives of Therapists' Lives. Adelaide: Dulwich Centre Publications.

WHO (World Health Organization) and Calouste Gulbenkian Foundation (2014) Social Determinants of Mental Health. Geneva: WHO.

Wilkinson, R. and Pickett, K. (2010) The Spirit Level: Why Equality is Better for Everyone. London: Penguin.

Winship, G. (2016) A meta-recovery framework: positioning the 'new recovery' movement and other recovery approaches. Journal of Psychiatric and Mental Health Nursing, 23(1): 66–73.

Worrall, L., Mather, K. and Seifert, R. (2010) Solving the labour problem among professional workers in the UK public sector: organisation change and performance management. Public Organization Review, 10(2): 117–137.

Zubin, J. and Spring, B. (1977) Vulnerability: a new view of schizophrenia. Journal of Abnormal Psychology, 86(2): 103–126.

Index

References to endnotes show both the
page number and the note number (231n3).